HOW TO CARE FOR YOUR PARENTS

A PRACTICAL GUIDE

TO ELDERCARE

R

HOW TO CARE FOR YOUR PARENTS

A PRACTICAL GUIDE TO

ELDERCARE

NORA JEAN LEVIN

W · W · NORTON & COMPANY

NEW YORK   LONDON

s: A Handbook for Adult Children

right © 1986 by Herb Gardner.

from this book, write to Permissions,
rk, NY 10110.

The text of this book is composed in 12.75 / 15 Perpetua, with the display set in Felix Titling.
Composition manufacturing by The Haddon Craftsmen, Inc.
Book design by Margaret M. Wagner.

Library of Congress Cataloging-in-Publication Data

Levin, Nora Jean.
How to care for your parents : a practical guide to eldercare / by Nora Jean Levin.
p.   cm.
Includes bibliographical references and index.
ISBN 0-393-03987-0.—ISBN 0-393-31526-6 (pbk.)
1. Aging parents—Care—United States—Handbooks, manuals, etc.   2. Adult
children—United States—Handbooks, manuals, etc. 3. Caregivers—United States—
Handbooks, manuals, etc. 4. Aged—Services for—United States.   I. Title.
HQ1063.6.L49 1997
306.874—dc20   96-20955
                                                                CIP

W. W. Norton & Company, Inc., 500 Fifth Avenue, New York, N.Y. 10110
http://www.wwnorton.com

W. W. Norton & Company Ltd., 10 Coptic Street, London WC1A 1PU

1 2 3 4 5 6 7 8 9 0

To the memory of
my beloved father, Hirsch Bieler,
my dear father-in-law Benjamin Levin,
and my mother-in-law supreme,
Beatrice Jackson Levin

CONTENTS

PREFACE

This book is about energy and attitude. It is also about saving time and money. It deals with life, not funerals, death, or dying. Ailing or aging parents still have a lot of living left to do. Their goal—*your* goal—is to help them do it. I have written this guide for adult children like me, who belong to the so-called "sandwich generation": caught between the demands of our own careers, midlife relationships, growing children, and the needs of aging parents. We want to do what is right—both for ourselves and for all those we love.

This book began with the increasing involvement of myself and my husband in decisions facing members of our own families. The need for increased involvement in our parents' care dawned slowly on us as they retired, became widowed, took ill. The inevitable losses they faced—of physical capabilities, loved ones, mental agility, a sense of purpose, or independence—initially prompted our sympathy and concern, but resulted in little direct action. Our participation increased when we began to see our parents having trouble managing not only their immediate financial affairs, but also *their* responsibilities toward their own aging parents and siblings.

I was quite confident in our ability to resolve issues quickly and effectively when we first volunteered our energy and time. As an information gatherer with careers in consumer advocacy, business, and education, I expected to draw on my past experience in planning, financial management, and decoding government mumbo jumbo to master these intertwined health and welfare issues. I was sure that what I didn't understand or couldn't read in the small print, my lawyer-spouse could. I aimed to research facts and collect information that would help our parents make better, more informed choices. I counted on familiar sources—libraries, telephone directories, bookstores, newspapers, reports, friends, computers. My husband tackled the forms and bills. He counted on his Washington regulatory credentials and bureaucratic skills.

How naive we were! Not only were the sources scattered, the information cumbersome, the codes cryptic, and the networks unfamiliar, but libraries, telephone directories, and bookstores proved to be poor hunting grounds. I soon found I didn't know how or where to look. I was digging in the wrong spots. I couldn't locate the proper categories; sometimes they just didn't exist. Magazines and newspapers helped. They had more information than books. But their articles were fragmented, leaving gaps as large as the holes they plugged. My husband found himself unprepared for the frustrating paperwork of medical claim forms, nursing home bills, and complex rules on Medicaid eligibility.

Our degrees and skills notwithstanding, we realized with

growing horror we could not be good consumers or effective advocates for our parents' care. We had landed in alien territory. We lacked maps to lead us through the labyrinth. Our ignorance and inexperience exaggerated such traditional barriers to care as cost, availability, transportation, and scheduling.

We found family decision making was impossible without timely, reliable information on available options. Access to such information was blocked because we were intimidated by the technical language and distracted by confusing terminology. Simple navigation tools and expert guides were hard to locate because of the lack of common reference standards and poor links between public and private, or formal and informal, networks of support services.

Finally, the very process of gathering information was clouded by the intense feelings our new role evoked. As confirmed by Louise Fradkin, co-founder of the self-help organization Children of Aging Parents, at a 1995 White House mini-conference on Aging:

> Caregivers are not good consumer advocates or sophisticated consumers. . . . The social service network, the medical terminology, that whole area is foreign to them when it comes to their parents. . . . Because layered on top of that is all the emotional trauma of suddenly being in a reverse situation—being the one to take care of a parent who was once your authority figure. Plus your family relationships. The emotional stress is phenomenal.

It turned out that a wealth of information on available health and support services was there—once we started asking the right questions of the right people. We gradually discovered a whole new group of experts. But even these experts were hard to find. They were poorly advertised to the general public. Instead their services were directed towards professional advisors scattered around the "health network," the "aging network," private voluntary groups, or community organizations. Their information was also aimed at our parents—not at us, their concerned children.

The specialists we found—lawyers, social workers, doctors, accountants, psychiatrists, financial planners, stockbrokers, bankers, occupational therapists, even morticians, and clergymen—all made valuable suggestions. They said, "Do this, do that. Beware of this. That will cost money. Above all, remember that, like crime, Medicare does not pay." But as months passed, assembling our recipe box of "coping strategies" became a complicated effort that diverted increasing amounts of personal and career time.

Then the real obstacle course began. To our surprise, we found that once we had the necessary information, defined our choices, and were ready to make decisions—our parents were often not ready or willing to act. Our timetables and persuasions dissolved in mutual frustration, sometimes in tears. Still, my husband and I found that as we learned what decisions needed to be made and what choices were available, we gained patience and reduced our own anxiety. And together with our parents we discovered options that opened avenues of hope, not roads to gloom or despair. That was crucial, since gloom seemed to be spreading.

Most important, we learned that the critical questions regarding care for our parents related to a shifting range of capabilities—ours as well as theirs. The less capable they became in certain areas, the more we needed to do—or arrange to have done. The more capable they were in other areas, the less assistance they needed. But all along that range—behind each key decision affecting our parents' independence, freedom of choice, and quality of life—lay numerous options and support services.

Each of these options had a cost. Some costs were modest, involving only small sums of money. Others involved pride or self-sufficiency. Some were so expensive they would impoverish even the rich. But all were available, where we had thought none existed.

We learned that parents needing personal care do not have to give up their home or their privacy and move in with their children—or into a nursing home. Many "healthcare" housing options now make it possible for parents to keep the comforts of home by adding needed support services.

We learned of catalogs filled with information about "assistive devices" and about supportive senior-citizen programs, from beepers to transportation, whose sole purpose is to help people live more independently. Not all were available (or called by the same name) everywhere, but there were dozens more than we had thought.

We learned that certain legal documents could preserve and carry out a parent's wishes, despite disability or incompetence. We discovered that programs like Medicare were not necessarily the "safety nets" we had assumed—and that new private insurance and community-based service plans were available to fill some of the holes. We learned that using the "information highway" on our home computer could dramatically expand our ability to find information, resources, and much-needed peer support—even after business hours.

Eventually we found that in caring for our parents we had gathered a bookful of knowledge about choices, support services, and useful tips that could help others on that path. This handbook is the result.

How to Care for Your Parents assumes you are "stepping in" for the first time. It introduces the main buzzwords, junctures, and pitfalls you will likely encounter in the process of caregiving. It assumes that while you and your parents understand some changes are necessary to plan for their future, you both may need help making these decisions. It also assumes you will need help figuring out what decisions to make.

This handbook offers a systematic approach for gathering important information. It identifies and organizes options for health and long-term care. Its premise is that for the welfare of your family, the best plans emerge from joint efforts.

ACKNOWLEDGMENTS

I first wrote *How to Care forYour Parents* in 1987 to share practical experience—and help other caregivers and their loved ones overwhelmed by these complex issues, information, and decisions. Because consumer education depends on access to reliable information on health and human services, and because access requires advance planning, I made special efforts to identify the barriers which make these tasks more difficult. In this revision, as with previous editions, I am grateful for the generously shared experiences, materials and expertise of the numerous friends, and practitioners and researchers in the aging field who promptly and thoroughly responded to my persistent requests. Thanks, among many others to:

Mildred Marmur, my agent, who first brought this book to Norton's attention; Amy Cherry, unflappable editor; Kate Barry, tenacious copy editor, without whom this book would not have come to be.

Denise Hussar, APPRISE, Pennsylvania Department of Aging; Michael Knipmeyer, HICP, George Washington University, Washington, D.C.; Priscilla Itscoitz, United Seniors Health Cooperative; Sara Aravanis and Bernice Hutchinson, National Association of State Units on Aging (NASUA); and

Eric Lang at HHS' Health Care Financing Administration (HCFA), for information about Health Insurance Counseling Programs.

Edward Hutman of Benefit Services, Inc., Reisterstown, Maryland for continuing updates on developments in long-term care insurance.

David Kane of Hyatt's Classic Residence, Bethesda, Maryland for an administrator's view of trends in assisted living.

Denise Franz of Medicaid statistics at HCFA for demystifying the statistics and clarifying actual Medicaid numbers and expenditures for the over-sixty-five population.

Louise Fradkin and Ed Madara for their pathbreaking work on caregiver Self-Help groups and the possibilities of Eldercare online. Mary Gardiner Jones for her commitment to a future where affordable telecommunications technology will bring computers to the world of home care.

Attorneys Janet Kuhn of McLean, Virginia, and Herb Semmel, Los Angeles, California and Patricia Nemour of the National Senior Citizens Law Center, Washington, D.C., who, by interview and writings, carefully detailed the repercussions of block grant proposals for Medicaid reform.

Georgia Sales of the Los Angeles InfoLine and the Alliance of Information and Referral Systems (AIRS) for her ongoing work bringing a common language and taxonomy to the human service arena.

Senior moving coordinators Donna Quinn Robbins of Oakland, California and Shannon McDonald of Alexandria, Virginia for their entrepreneurial work bringing order and relieving the stress of moving. Interior Design consultant Irma Dopkin, who combines personal with professional zeal in the concepts of universal design. Linda Sterthous of the Partnership Group, Blue Bell, Pennsylvania, for updating older material.

Tom Poole of Senior.Com; Steve Gurney of the *Guide to Retirement Living;* Jeff Finn of the SPRY Foundation and Compuserve's Retirement Living Forum; Bruce Craig at the Administration on Aging; Joyce Post, librarian of the Philadelphia Geriatric Center, are each in their way doing pioneer work both opening up the Internet as a resource for Seniors and in categorizing the work of others so seekers can find it. And the wonderful telephone technicians at Clarknet, without whom I never would have gotten online.

Mary Lee Di Spirito, Mary Beth Franklin, and Tania Haftel (my sister), were kind enough to read and critique draft material. Mary Lee is one of the many caregivers I've met over the past few years whose from-the-trenches opinions I value so highly. Mary Beth Franklin is a gifted journalist who has done important work communicating eldercare information to a mass audience.

Dear friends Anne McCormick, Audrey Wolf, Johanna Neuman, Paris Suzanne Singer, and Seth Shulman, have been my caregiver role models teaching courage, compassion, unfailing energy, good spirits, and the ability to work the system, while juggling work and family responsibilities.

Susan Schneider, Jane Plakias, and Steve Eastham, for being such patient listeners and lifelines.

My mother, Anna Bieler, who never ceases to amaze me with her sharp insight and "naked truth" perspective on aging. She keeps me honest.

My husband, Michael, genius in making the obtuse clear,

who has somehow maintained our enthusiasm for this unending project, and always found time to read its reappearing drafts.

Sons Jeremy and Dan for their forbearance, and for not asking more than once each week when I would get a "real job."

Finally, to Sam, who as a sled-dog can't quite read, but is always ready to go to the park and have a nice walk, for knowing exactly when it's time to stop work and start play.

HOW TO CARE FOR YOUR PARENTS

A PRACTICAL GUIDE

TO ELDERCARE

INTRODUCTION: STEPPING IN

WHEN DO YOU STEP IN?

When do you step in to help your parents? Usually when you least expect it:

- You get a midnight call from a stranger, reporting that your father is in the emergency room for surgery.

- You get a chatty letter from your mother, with a bombshell planted between gossip. By the way, she says, dad went to renew his driver's license, flunked his eye exam, and had his license revoked. Since your parents live far from public transportation and have difficulty walking, they are in trouble.

- One of your parents' neighbors pulls you aside and suggests gently or bluntly that despite your parents' bright attitude, arthritis (or heart disease or depression) is taking a heavy toll. The neighbor says your parents don't want to burden you, but someone ought to say something.

- During a rare four-day visit to your house, while you race between delivering juice to your son's soccer game and picking up the cake for your daughter's birthday party, your increasingly nervous mother breaks down during the car ride—your first moment alone together—and admits that she is very unhappy with her life, that it is all just "too much." She feels terrible about forgetting all the time, "can't seem to keep up anymore," and "doesn't know what to do."

These examples occur in dozens of variations, all leading to the same conclusion: Your parents need you—now.

The most important response is to understand what has just happened. Namely, you have reached that point when it is necessary to take action. The crisis itself may pass—emergencies always do—but the problem will not go away. Your parents have reached a stage where they need help, and you are it. No matter how inconvenient this may be for you, you must start providing the emotional, physical, legal, and financial support that is required. What you face is not really an emergency, but a *condition:* a whole new set of circumstances you will need to address seriously over time.

The sooner you accept this condition the better off you will be. So make yourself a cup of coffee, or wash the car, or go for a long jog, or a birdwalk, or shopping, and get a grip on yourself. Initially you may feel incompetent, over-whelmed, and trapped. Conflicting reactions of love, sadness, guilt, anxiety, resentment, anger, or inadequacy need to be sorted out. You knew the day was coming, but so soon? It isn't fair. Whether parents' conditions deteriorate rapidly or slowly, you are in for the long haul. Coping means recog-nizing this and dealing with the situation in the most practical, sensible, efficient—and most caring—manner possible. This will be best for your parents and you.

THE ELDERLY POPULATION

It may be some comfort to know you are not alone. Many of your friends are facing the same hard questions and decisions.

In 1900 the average American died at forty-seven. By 1987 the age rose to seventy-four. Today anyone who lives past fifty can expect to reach eighty-three. In 1900 there were three million Americans sixty-five or older. By 1996 there were over thirty-three million—more than 12 percent of our population. In fact, Americans over eighty-five are now the fastest growing part of the population. Those over 100 are the second fastest growing segment.

This explains why the topic of "eldercare" crops up so frequently when those of us over forty get together. And why, at some gatherings, it is the only subject we discuss. Contrary to popular belief, most care for the elderly is not provided in hospitals or other institutions, but by family members in private households.

As you have probably noticed, the majority of senior citizens are women. Studies show that:

- In 1994, there were three women for every man age sixty-five or older;

- Women now live almost eight years longer than men, and are the main users of long-term care;

- In 1990 nearly half of all older women were widows; there were five times as many widows as widowers;

- Women comprise three of every four elderly persons living below the poverty line;

- The number of elderly women living alone has doubled in the last fifteen years;

- Four of every five nursing home residents are women.

In other words, modern medicine has prolonged life—but it has not guaranteed health. More than four-fifths of Americans over sixty-five have at least one chronic health problem. Whether they suffer from conditions like arthritis (where the body is diminished but the mind is intact), or Alzheimer's disease (where the body stays strong but the mind weakens), older peoples' abilities to perform such basic daily tasks as dressing, eating, bathing, voiding, walking, and getting out of bed gradually decrease. So do their abilities to manage shopping, cooking, housework, yard chores, handling money, and driving. Today Americans sixty-five to seventy-six often remain active and independent. But from then on, they are twenty times more likely to need personal assistance than those under sixty-five.

There is some good news in these numbers. While chronic illness among older people is common, four out of five seniors over sixty-five are "functionally healthy." This means they are doing mostly what they choose, helped by miracles of modern medicine such as corneal implants, open-heart surgery, medication, and devices ranging from pacemakers to artificial hips. A University of Miami survey of Americans over eighty-five found that only one out of three is in a nursing home. The others are still out in the community. Most of these people lived in their own homes as heads of a household. A few still worked for a living. Over half were fit enough to use public transportation. Though one in six needed financial assistance, twice that number were financially comfortable.

As adult children you will need to understand—not minimize or exaggerate—your parents' limitations. You will also need to disconnect the prejudice that links age with automatic incapacity. As you go about this task, accept parents' chronic conditions as permanent, not aberrations to be ignored or overattended. The focus is less on cure than on health, management, and coping. This is the time to be grown up—not resentful, hostile, or tearful. You have got to think positively. Your attitude will make an enormous difference in how your parents live the rest of their lives. So will theirs.

Look around. It is obvious that age or debility are not the only criteria defining quality of life. Ailments notwithstanding, a person may be more optimistic and vigorous at eighty-five than someone healthy and fifty. Attitude towards life is enormously important in the ability to cope.

Getting involved in the care of your parents does not mean taking over all aspects of their lives or physically taking care of them. Instead you need to start the process of framing questions and helping make choices affecting their lives and yours. To do this effectively requires cooperation and organization. You will need to learn what resources parents have on hand, what outside resources are available, and how to use them. Your job will be complicated because you will need to figure out what is best for everyone—not only for your parents, but for yourself and members of your own family.

WHAT ARE THE MAJOR TASKS?

The major tasks you and your parents will face in preparing for a future where they may need some support from you are:

- Locating and evaluating resources needed to make informed choices;
- Planning for legal and financial incapacities;
- Understanding and managing income and expenses;
- Arranging for long-term care.

To make sound decisions, you must grapple with the technical, physical, and emotional aspects of these tasks. For example, you will need to:

- Assess your parents' various needs and the capabilities of the whole family unit;
- Collect information on how to address those specific needs;
- Divide responsibilities between parents, siblings, relatives, friends, neighbors, and other sources of support;
- Reach for help from outside information experts and community backup services;
- Investigate using new technologies and adapting available devices to maintain parents' independence or reduce their functional impairments; and

· Repeat all this six months later, because circumstances usually change. Often they worsen. But more often than you'd think, they improve.

HOW MUCH SHOULD YOU DO?

How much should you do? There is no job description on caring for parents. Every family does it differently. You may be great at emotional support but awful as a financial manager. You may be a wonderful comparison shopper, but freeze at telephone calls. You may be a super information gatherer with piles of files on various services, but an impatient hands-on caregiver. Your weakness may be your brother's or sister's strength, or you may share weaknesses and strengths with your siblings and need some outside help. Help can take the form of hiring a medical claims service, or paying for in-house services, or finding adult day care programs. It can come from the private sector, the local church or hospital, or other community-based support programs. When all is said and done, your role as your parents' manager, helper, shopper, sympathetic friend, or personal hand-holder will be defined and shaped by your love, your capabilities, and your own unique resources, as well as theirs.

The material in this book may be unfamiliar. Its information, warnings, and tips may seem overwhelming. But do not be discouraged or alarmed. There is nothing wrong with you. Because so many new topics need to be touched on, it takes some time just to map the terrain. So skim the book, see what you need most, and start there. When you have gotten a grip on that, go on to sections that address other topics that match your needs.

Part One, "Getting Organized," shows you a way to assemble information your parents will need to make responsible decisions about their future. The first task is to identify their specific needs. The second is to gather and consolidate all their "personal records" so you have a snapshot of where they stand. Third, you'll prepare a "Financial Profile" to evaluate how to meet increased costs of care. The fourth task is to use multiple tools—the telephone book, workplace employee assistance programs, and home computer links with the World Wide Web and Internet—to find what support networks and community resources are available to help.

"Gathering Resources," the second part of the book, is divided into two sections. The first is a primer on community resources. The second section introduces the possibilities and pitfalls of finding eldercare resources online. It surveys the major ramps of the Internet, offers pointers to finding information, and details how specific sites may be of use. The decisions you and your parents make will be based on the groundwork you do in Parts One and Two.

In Part Three "Making Decisions," additional steps are outlined that can help you arrange for your parents' care and welfare. To help you understand and better evaluate information affecting their choices, "Taking Preventive Measures" discusses insurance and other protections against "worst-case" catastrophe involving incapacity and impoverishment. "Securing Safety and Welfare" focuses on how to make your parents' home safer and more comfortable, and illustrates the range of new possibilities for improved at-home care. From smaller apartments to nursing homes to moving in with you, "Looking at Housing Options" describes the current choices and how to go about downsizing, a process useful for any household move.

And finally, Part Four, "Juggling Obligations," highlights the emotional pitfalls you will encounter as caregivers. It also offers some advice on how to avoid them, or climb back out as quickly as possible.

PART ONE

GETTING
ORGANIZED

Getting organized to help care for your parents is a multi-step process that will require time and energy as well as sensitivity and patience. After all, the tables are turning and your parents may now be looking to you for additional support and guidance—even if they are reluctant to acknowledge the fact. It takes time for both of you to adjust to this new situation. But there are rewards. And getting organized can help reduce both anxiety and stress.

By gathering information included in this section, you can lower the first barrier that blocks your parents' ability to retain their independence, safety, and quality of life. To assess available options for your parents' care it helps to know their strengths and weaknesses, their needs, and the available help. The more complete the information you collect, the clearer your picture for planning and evaluating choices. And the sooner that picture is assembled, the greater the savings in time and money. Your aim is to help your parents understand that it is in their interest to work with you now to avoid future regrets. You will need their help to gather three kinds of information:

· Information on parents' specific care needs.

· Personal information that you probably do not have, such as parents' social security numbers, insurance coverage, health records, and financial status. The resulting profile of their legal, financial, and medical status will be crucial for numerous decisions.

· Community resource information on services and programs currently available in your parents' community and (if you live elsewhere) in your own. As you start to dig, you will discover a web of health, human service, and aging networks offering such support as transportation, home healthcare, and counseling. You may also discover that the networks are poorly integrated and you are the only one connecting its links.

To gather the necessary information requires pulling together documents, collecting data, and preparing lists. In fact, as you will see, the process involves following twenty-two simple steps and preparing nine different document records. With these records in hand, you will have a much clearer picture of your parents' affairs. This knowledge, combined with information on available resources in the community, will become the basis for advance planning.

However, despite your good intentions, your parents may not welcome questions about their personal documents, health conditions, or ability to manage finances. Your concern may seem heavy-handed or strike sensitive spots. Face it, your parents may not be interested in changing the way they live; few people are. They may not want you, or anyone else, to meddle in their affairs. Expect some resistance. In fact, expect a lot of resistance. This common reaction may have more to do with parents' personal pride, family relationships, or past coping patterns than recent events. On the other hand, it may stem from mental or emotional problems. But it may also stem from a healthy feeling that your parents are still in charge of their lives, have not asked for your help, and do not want it.

Fair enough. You do not need to know all the details, especially if your parents are still managing their personal finances and are generally in control. But once you explain that gathering basic information and having it readily available will make it easier to collect insurance benefits, receive retirement pensions, or sell property, your parents will probably move faster than expected to arrange their affairs on their own and take you (or another person they trust) into their confidence. Further, your parents need to understand that should they become sick or incapacitated, no one—neither you nor an alternate responsible party—can help them without certain documents and information.

As for the parallel task—tapping into health and aging service networks—get used to the idea you will need to talk to a lot of strangers, people who can advise you on the kinds of assistance and long-term options available for your parents. Your precision in framing key questions to these "providers"—questions on healthcare, housing, finances, transportation, or home services—will improve the quality of their response. You won't believe how many new contacts you'll make, and how much you'll learn.

If you are lucky, organizing personal and financial materials will be relatively painless. You may even discover your parents already use community support systems. But don't count on it. Very few households are so well managed that each important document or telephone number is readily available and up to date. Like everyone else, older people disregard details. They leave insurance forms piled on the desk or ignore complicated letters from banks, brokers, or pension funds. And as frustrated providers are well aware, knowing about a service and actually using it are very different matters.

Chances are you will achieve many of your organizing goals quickly. But don't be surprised if others take a longer time to complete. Searching for one key document or working through one maze-like bank record or pension file may take months. Still, it is necessary to do the most thorough job you can. As you will see later, the more complete the information you collect about their health, social support, and finances, the more options you will uncover and the more choices you will have to help your parents make good decisions. Moreover, delay is costly in terms of time, money, and stress. So you should get started now before the next emergency hits.

These twenty-two steps are designed to help you assemble information so it can be efficiently used. That will speed up the process when you need to see a lawyer, evaluate housing, or deal with urgent healthcare choices.

Getting organized may not be easy. But if you go about it diligently, you will be amazed how far you and your parents will get. Working together, you will track down important documents, gaining a better understanding of their contents. You will identify some areas that need attending and combine or simplify many routine chores.

Just as important, you will have gained knowledge about the many outside resources available in your parents' community. You will have a much better idea how and where you and your parents can "plug into the system" to arrange for support.

Remember, there is no reason to wait until you complete every step within each task before going on to the next. If you hit obstacles in one area (working out the details of a will, for example), pursue another while you work the first one through. Move at the speed and in the order that is best for you and your parents.

And when this phase is complete, you will be much better prepared to make some decisions.

IDENTIFYING PROBLEMS AND NEEDS

This is the heart of your job. It is painful to watch those we love suffer the indignities of not being able to perform routine tasks. Your parents may be very stubborn, waiting until the last minute to call for help, then plunging everyone into a crisis situation. Stepping back to identify issues and specific needs so parents can retain their independence and improve their quality of life *before* a real emergency is a key step in organizing for care. And preparing this first list is a good way to open a dialogue about your concerns.

STEP 1—IDENTIFY PROBLEMS AND NEEDS

The process of identifying "care needs" for your parents can occur informally or formally. Either way, the items you identify will change over time. This process can involve many people inside or outside the family. Since your concern has already committed you to stepping in, now is the time to sharpen your focus. Once you do this, you can break identified problems down into smaller, more manageable units.

For example, if your mother is socially isolated because she no longer drives, she needs transportation in order to be with other people. Or perhaps she should move closer to activities. If her vision or hearing or memory are failing, these conditions will likely have profound effects on her emotional health. Technology in the form of assistive devices and home modification, or a trained pet to serve as eyes or ears, or counseling and home care, all can help her.

Taking the following list (adapted from the *Care Management Guide, Caregivers in the Workplace,* American Association of Retired Persons, 1987) as a guide, you can get started on your own particulars:

My relative . . .

__ needs to get out of the house
__ can manage light housecleaning but needs help with heavy tasks
__ is grieving over the death of a loved one
__ doesn't eat regularly
__ shouldn't be left home alone
__ pays insufficient attention to money matters
__ needs special services for physical limitations
__ needs twenty-four-hour supervision

When you finish your list, review each item with your parents (and whoever else is involved in their care). Next, prioritize the list by scale ("this is a big/little problem") and urgency ("we've got to do something NOW/can wait until later").

As you will see, other sections of this handbook will help you plan for long-term care, show you how to preserve your parent's wishes in the event of incapacity, and help you to find backup services to meet their needs. But isolating the specific problems is a key first step in developing plans to help you achieve your goals. The purpose of this preliminary review is to see what can be done to help promote your loved ones' independence, safety, and satisfaction with their lifestyle. The information you will collect in the following sections will help you identify the matching resources.

CREATING A PERSONAL PROFILE

Steps 2–9 help you identify, locate and collect the information you and your parents will need to create a personal profile. By following this part you will prepare lists in four general categories:

- Personal Documents

- Medical History

- Personal Support System

- Financial Resources and Obligations

STEP 2—MAKE A PERSONAL DOCUMENTS LIST

Every person acquires personal documents as he or she goes through life. These usually include a birth certificate, a passport, a marriage certificate (or several, along with divorce decrees), a Social Security card, and a pension fund membership. None of us has the same documents because we lead such different lives. One person may acquire three divorce decrees and title to twelve houses. Another may never marry or own property.

You need to make customized lists relevant to your parents' lives. To do this, use the list below, crossing out items that do not pertain to your parents. You can ask your parents to do this, or do it together with them—not on the telephone, but face to face in their home.

Review the customized list below. In the "Status" column put a check next to items your parents have and can locate, an X by those items your parents have but cannot find: and a star ★ by those items your parents ought to have but don't—such as wills or a lost Social Security card.

PERSONAL DOCUMENTS

_____

DATE

STATUS	PERSONAL DOCUMENTS	LOCATION
_____	Birth certificate	_____
_____	Adoption papers	_____
_____	Passport	_____
_____	Marriage certificate	_____
_____	Divorce/Separation decrees	_____
_____	Naturalization papers	_____
_____	Military records	_____
_____	Cemetery deed	_____
_____	Funeral instructions	_____
_____	Income tax returns—prior years	_____
_____	Income tax return—current year	_____
_____	Gift and gift tax records	_____
_____	Estate/inheritance tax returns	_____
_____	House deeds and titles	_____
_____	Mortgages	_____
_____	Auto titles	_____
_____	Durable power of attorney	_____
_____	Alternate power of attorney	_____

STATUS	PERSONAL DOCUMENTS	LOCATION
_____	Advance directives:	_____
	___ Living will	_____
	___ Medical (or healthcare) power of attorney	_____
_____	Will	_____
_____	Living trust agreement	_____
_____	Letters of instruction in case of death	_____
_____	Medicare card	_____
_____	Medicaid card	_____
_____	Private health insurance policy	_____
_____	Long-term care insurance policy	_____
_____	Life insurance policy	_____
_____	Disability insurance policy	_____
_____	Automobile insurance policy	_____
_____	Homeowner/Apartment insurance policy	_____

Step 3—Preview the List and Locate the Documents

Now you need to locate all the checked items. Although most of these documents should be in special safekeeping, you will probably find them everywhere. Your parents may have important papers locked in a safe deposit box in their bank, or in a shoe box in a closet, or tucked away as mementos in scrapbooks. Some may be stuffed in desk drawers or filing cabinets. Some may be in the attics of distant relatives, or the files of present or former lawyers, stockbrokers, or accountants.

Next find or replace all the papers marked X. Tracking down these papers may take hours or weeks. If one is missing and you need to replace it, be prepared for frustrating phone calls and bureaucratic run-arounds. On the bright side, this hunt for parents' personal documents may yield precious bits of family history as well as vital information. For example, the simple question "Do you have a cemetery plot?" might turn up the fact that Uncle Joe is the only one who knows. Calling him, you discover the name of the cemetery and the plot's location, along with the fact that he bought two plots—for himself and your mother—after a glamorous niece you never heard of died during a 1942 flu epidemic. If your parents, like mine, were born in other countries, their explanations of why they do not have birth certificates may be worth recording.

As you find each document, note its location on the list or add a ★ showing you need it. Durable power of attorney and advance directives (instructions for healthcare, including a medical power of attorney and living will) will most likely be in the ★ category. They are legal delegation-of-authority documents, items your parents will absolutely need should they ever have a terminal or debilitating illness. These documents protect your parents right to have family or others they choose make end-of-life decisions concerning their care should they be unable to act on their own (see p. 187 for more information).

STEP 4—REVIEW THE DOCUMENTS AND NOTE ITEMS FOR FUTURE ACTION

Once you have the documents, review each one carefully. You may discover that certain papers (your father's will, for example) are outdated. Or you may discover that a key document is up-to-date but inaccurate. For example, your mother's Social Security card may have the wrong first or last name on it.

The following are a few sample questions to ask during your review to identify gaps that require later action.

Questions:

1. Do your parents have a will? When was it last reviewed? Is it current on its provisions, beneficiaries, executor, and other arrangements? Does it address the simultaneous death of a spouse? Is it in accord with current state law?

2. What arrangements have been made should one or both parents lose competence to handle their affairs? Who will handle their money? If your father designates your mother, has she ever balanced a checkbook or prepared a tax return?

3. What preferences do your parents have about medical treatment should they become incompetent?

4. Have parents signed durable power of attorney forms allowing others to make healthcare and property decisions for their benefit? Who have they chosen as their "proxy" if they can't act for themselves? Have they drafted living wills? Are these documents valid if they live in one state but receive medical care in another?

5. Who will care for other aged or inform relatives for whom your parents are responsible?

6. What insurance protection exists for catastrophic illness or long-term custodial care? Are your parents overinsured—or undercovered?

7. Do they carry an emergency card in their wallet with insurance and proxy information, along with the names of their doctors and emergency contacts, and brief medical data including medications and dosages?

STEP 5—STORE THE DOCUMENTS

Now you have gathered and reviewed parents' personal documents and brought them up to date (making a note to fill gaps as you go on). Your next task, whatever storage system your parents use, is to learn where key documents are stored and how you can retrieve them in an emergency. This is a good time to gather documents together and store them in a single safe place.

• For documents stored in a bank vault, have your parents request a "signature card" with your name for the bank's file. This authorization allows you to gain entry, should the need arise.

· For documents parents keep at home, make sure you know precisely where they are. If any are under lock and key, write down the combination of the lock or where parents keep the key.

STEP 6—COMPILE A MEDICAL HISTORY FILE

Your parents need to consolidate and have readily available their complete medical history should they decide to move from one city to another to be closer to you; or stay in the same city, but experience a worsening health condition which requires a different level of treatment; or apply for Social Security disability benefits. In this instance, they will have to report on dates they were seen by doctors as well as the different doctors they may have consulted.

The Caregiver's Guide suggests creating a medical information "super-file" to help you handle such situations. For each chronic condition it recommends gathering information about the condition itself, the doctors who last treated it, and the various tests performed and medications prescribed.

If your mom is like mine, by the eighth or ninth decade, her list of body parts needing regular attention or repair will be long indeed. The following is a list of fourteen conditions that affect older people. You will probably recognize more than a few. So, starting with religion, blood type, known or suspected drug allergies (if any), and recent surgeries, customize a medical history list from the guide below.

MEDICAL HISTORY

_____

DATE

RELIGION _____

BLOOD TYPE _____

KNOWN DRUG ALLERGIES _____

RECENT SURGERY _____

CONDITION* _____

1. Memory and thinking problems such as dementia

2. Neurologic disorders such as Parkinson's disease and stroke

3. Mood disorders such as anxiety and depression

4. Skin conditions including pressure ulcers and shingles

5. Joints/Muscles and bones including back, feet, knees, osteoporosis

6. Head, neck, and sensory conditions including hearing, dental, and thyroid

7. Heart and circulation conditions

8. Blood disorders

9. Lung and breathing problems

10. Digestive disorders including swallowing difficulties, constipation

11. Nutrition concerns including malnutrition and obesity

12. Bladder, urinary, and kidney conditions

13. Sexual concerns such as gynecologic disorders and prostate problems

14. Other conditions such as cancer, diabetes, pain, sleep problems, walking problems, and falls

DOCTOR   ADDRESS/PHONE

TESTS   MEDICATIONS   DATE

DOCTOR   ADDRESS/PHONE

TESTS   MEDICATIONS   DATE

DOCTOR   ADDRESS/PHONE

TESTS   MEDICATIONS   DATE

DOCTOR   ADDRESS/PHONE

TESTS   MEDICATIONS   DATE

---

*List of conditions adapted from chapter headings of Mark E. Williams, M.D., American Geriatric Society, *Complete Guide to Aging and Health* (Harmony Books, New York), 1995.

· If you start from scratch, and your parents are vague on details, a time-saving tip is to ask to see their pile of Medicare "EOBs" (Explanation of Medicare Part B Benefits). The benefits statement, headed by a bold "THIS IS NOT A BILL," lists the name of the physician, the date of the office visit, and the procedures performed. Sort this pile by doctor name to give you a quick chronological medical review of recent treatment. For your own sanity, ignore explanations of charges and Medicare approved rates, at least for now.

· You can also contact their pharmacist for more information on medications and frequency of dosage (see Step 37, pp. 91, 198).

STEP 7—MAKE AN UPDATED LIST OF YOUR PARENT'S PERSONAL SUPPORT SYSTEM

Now that you have collected this information, keep going. It is time to consolidate, update, and create a list incorporating the names and telephone numbers of people your parents rely on for medical, legal, financial, religious, and personal support. Start with the basic information. Then customize the following list for your own parents:

PERSONAL SUPPORT SYSTEM

DATE _____

Name_____

Date of birth_____

Social Security number_____

Driver's license_____

Medicare number_____

Medicaid number_____

Health insurance policy number_____

SUPPORT	NAME	PHONE	ADDRESS
Emergency contact #1			
Emergency contact #2			
Relatives			
Friends			
Neighbors			
Chore/Household helpers			
Front desk—*(if they live in an apartment building)*			
Emergency room			
—Hospital choice			
Ambulance service			
Taxi service			
Poison control			

SUPPORT	NAME	PHONE	ADDRESS
Doctors			
Pharmacist			
Visiting nurse/Physical therapists			
Social service workers			
Police			
Fire department			
Church/Synagogue			
Pastor/Rabbi/Priest			
Attorney			
Banker			
Investment advisor			
Stockbroker			
Insurance agents			
Accountant			
Guardian or conservator			
Trustee			

If they are able, your parents should prepare this list. If not, do it together with them, since most of the information comes from their address books, correspondence, or scraps of paper kept near the telephone or on their refrigerator. After the list is done, follow up with a call to the listed insurance agents, stockbrokers, or lawyers to doublecheck telephone numbers and addresses. You may learn that names or addresses have changed as advisors moved, retired, or died. If so, ask how parents' records can be transferred or who has them now. Addresses and phone numbers of neighbors, friends, or relatives may also shift with the seasons, as retirees follow the sun. The list above suggests the kinds of people to include.

STEP 8—MAKE A FINANCIAL RESOURCES AND OBLIGATIONS LIST

This fourth list concerns money. Since the cost of managing parents' care may be a priority for years to come, stretching income to meet expenses will be a large part of the overall effort. This financial responsibility may not rest exclusively on your shoulders. But you certainly will be involved.

Besides, whoever has primary responsibility should know at a glance what resources your parents have at their disposal, and what debts or other obligations exist. In an emergency, easy access to this information can be invaluable, as a good friend of mine learned. Her dad was a World War II veteran. He lived in Florida with his wife on a modest income. While visiting her home in Washington, D.C., he unexpectedly suffered a debilitating stroke, needing not only extended hospitalization but sustained custodial care. Searching for a local nursing home my friend learned that the veterans' hospital was an excellent facility with available space. Because she had the specifics of her father's veterans' status, along with the telephone number of a contact person at her fingertips, she was able to place him in the VA facility, saving precious days, reducing unbearable stress, and avoiding financial catastrophe for the family.

Similarly, should such need arise in your family, having account information as well as contact/phone numbers of insurance agents, bankers, investment advisors, and pension plan representatives will help you move or shift funds quickly.

Beyond contacts and telephone numbers, getting a handle on finances by making lists of separate and joint resources and obligations is a necessary step *for everyone*—parents who have retired and adjusted comfortably to fixed incomes; parents approaching retirement; or parents whose expenses outstrip available resources.

This checklist has two parts. Part A itemizes by category, account numbers, location, and contact person. Part B provides detailed information on the income, expenses, and account balances for each item in Part A. This task is time-consuming. So begin with Part A, leaving Part B for later (see page 46).

FINANCIAL RESOURCES AND OBLIGATIONS—Part A

_____
DATE

BANKS

	INSTITUTION	ADDRESS	ACCOUNT	CONTACT/ PHONE
Checking				
Savings				
Money market				

INSURANCE

TYPE	COMPANY	ADDRESS	ACCOUNT	CONTACT/ PHONE
Whole life				
Term				
Annuity (tax-sheltered)				
Annuity (single-premium)				
Accident				
Other				

PENSION AND RETIREMENT PLANS

TYPE	ACCOUNT	BENEFIT	BENEFICIARY	CONTACT/ PHONE
Civil service				
Veterans' benefit				
Foreign service				

Type	Account	Benefit	Beneficiary	Contact/ Phone
Railroad retirement				
Fraternal organizations				
Other				

INVESTMENTS

Type	Location	Account	Contact/ Phone
Treasury notes			
Savings bonds			
CDs			
Bonds			
Stocks			
Mutual funds			
Other			

TAX-DEFERRED INVESTMENTS AND SHELTERS

Location	Address	Account	Contact/ Phone
Limited partnerships			
IRA			
Keogh			
Profit sharing			
Pension plans			
Other			

REAL ESTATE AND BUSINESS INTERESTS

TYPE	ADDRESS	INTEREST	LOCATION	CONTACT/ PHONE
Partnerships				
Business				
Real estate property				

VALUABLES

TYPE	LOCATION
Jewelry	
Paintings	
Other art objects	
Coin/Stamps	
Silverware	
Antiques	
Rare books	
Other valuables	

DEBTS

TYPE	LENDER	ADDRESS	PAYMENTS	DATES DUE	CONTACT/ PHONE
Mortgages					
Auto loans					
Credit cards					
Personal debts					
Other					

This information will come from many scattered sources. Again, customize the list to suit your parents' situation. While doing so, keep reminding your parents that while you are sensitive to their sense of financial privacy, this list *involves no actual figures.* Your parents may not wish to share the actual amounts with you. That is their privilege. All you really need to know is where these records are located, and how you or someone they trust can reach these records to act on your parents' behalf if necessary.

Depending on their capability, either offer them the master list to complete, or, working with your parent, go ahead and fill in the information together. In a perfect world, these records would be filed neatly in a drawer at parents' fingertips, or stored with other important papers in the bank. But you may need to do a little digging through piles of empty envelopes and years of bank statements. For example, you may need to track down account numbers, or carefully review a home insurance policy for a list of "scheduled" valuables. Do what you must to complete this list, paying close attention to the location of records, phone numbers, and contacts. You will need them later. *This is a vital document.*

STEP 9—DUPLICATE AND DISTRIBUTE THE FOUR LISTS

Congratulations! You have done quite a research job. Starting with identifying needs, you have listed your parents' Personal Documents, Medical History, Personal Support System, and Financial Resources and Obligations. Now tidy them up, and make several copies for your parents. Encourage them to send relevant copies to your siblings or other close family members, the family lawyer, primary physician, and executor of their wills. And, of course, keep a few handy for yourself, should the need arise.

Urge your parents to keep their Personal Support List readily available. However, the Financial Resources and Obligations List should be stored with other key documents.

CREATING A FINANCIAL PROFILE

Much of the stress of caring for parents has cold cash at its root. To deny or ignore this is to fool yourself. Either your parents have the resources to care for themselves, or they don't. If there is plenty of money, but its manager dies and the surviving spouse cannot or will not manage it, someone must. If there is not enough money and your parents must depend on outside sources of income or services, someone must identify and pursue those areas of potential support. That someone is you.

Your parents overall goals are peace of mind, independence, and the security to enjoy their final years. Key financial objectives to reach these goals include preserving income, maintaining self-sufficiency, protecting against catastrophic illness, reducing taxes, and providing for heirs.

In Steps 10–15, you and your parents will master their financial position and see how closely it matches their goals. In Step 19, you can take that profile to the experts to see what they suggest in planning for the future.

Parents' capabilities and desires for privacy will determine how personally involved you get in these tasks. Your approach is important. You will want to keep them focused on the advantages of consolidating important financial information into an "at-a-glance" format. But whether or not parents want to share the details with you at this point, someone they trust should know what is coming in, what is going out, and the relation between the two.

For purposes of this handbook, let's assume your parents have no accountant and hate numbers, so the pleasure of this task is yours. To save money and time, add up the numbers. The figures do not have to be exact. But there should be reasonable estimates for each category. The bankers, lawyers, accountants, insurance agents, investment counselors, social workers, benefits advisors, and financial planners you and your parents may later ask for advice will base their recommendations on figures in the statements you will prepare.

The Financial Profile consists of four documents:

- A resources and obligations list with dollar values

- A statement of yearly income and expenses

- A statement of monthly income and expenses

- A net worth statement

Step 10—Complete a Financial Inventory

This document supplements the Resources and Obligations List completed in Step 8. Your parents' command of and control over their finances will determine whether this material is easy or difficult to assemble. But even if it is difficult because you are starting from scratch, and they hold their securities in a safe deposit box and not at a brokerage house, once it is assembled it will be relatively simple to update. For example, fixed amounts will not change, and only recent transactions and account balances will need revisions:

FINANCIAL RESOURCES AND OBLIGATIONS—Part B

_____

DATE

CASH ACCOUNTS

NAME	CURRENT VALUE	INCOME
Checking		
Savings		
Money market		

TAXABLE INVESTMENTS

TYPE	MATURITY	YIELD	INCOME	PURCHASE DATE	PURCHASE PRICE
Savings bonds					
CDs					
Treasury notes					
Bonds					
Stocks					
Mutual funds					
Other					

TAX-DEFERRED INVESTMENTS AND SHELTERS

TYPE	CURRENT VALUE	INCOME	DATES PAYABLE
Limited partnerships			
Annuity (tax sheltered)			
IRA accounts			

Type	Current Value	Income	Dates Payable
Keogh accounts			
Profit sharing plans			
Pension plans			
Other			

TAX-FREE INVESTMENTS

Type	Maturity	Interest	Income	Dates Due
Mutual funds				
Municipal bonds				
Other				

REAL PROPERTY

Type	Appraised Value
Real estate	
Valuables	

INSURANCE

	Face Value	Cash Value	Insured	Owner	Beneficiary
Whole life					
Term					
Other					

DEBTS

Type	Lender	Amount	Dates Due
Mortgages			
Auto loans			
Credit cards			
Personal debts			
Other			

STEP 11—COMPLETE A STATEMENT OF MONTHLY INCOME AND EXPENSES

In Step 12 you will prepare a Statement of Yearly Income and Expenses. It will be easy to do this once you have prepared an income and expense statement for each month of the year. The monthly record shows the blips and dips when income exceeds expenses (or vice versa). When you total the numbers, you will quickly see where your parents' cash flow needs adjusting.

For instance, suppose a yearly annuity check from your mother's pension arrives in January. Before she races to invest this chunk of "extra income" in a long-term CD or tax-free bond—effectively locking away the cash for five, ten, or more years—it is important to know that in April her estimated tax payments are due and she faces a large insurance premium. Or suppose your dad lives in an "assisted-living facility" whose monthly rentals now exceed his pension and retirement checks. Spreading dividend, annuity, or investment payments over the four quarters of the year, or having them distributed monthly, may help make more funds available as needed. Until you see where and when income is needed, you cannot tell whether juggling distribution dates makes sense.

It should not take long to complete this form. If your parents have lived on a fixed income and managed their money for a long time, don't be surprised if they can rattle off their major monthly expenses by heart.

MONTHLY INCOME AND EXPENSE STATEMENT

_____
DATE

A. INCOME

TAXABLE	HUSBAND	WIFE	JOINT
Wages, salaries			
Other compensation			
Interest/Investment			
Rental or business income			
Social Security			
Pensions			
IRA/Keogh			
Annuity			
Rent			
Royalties			
Trust			
Other			

TAX-FREE

Bonds			
Mutual funds			
Portion of Social Security			

B. EXPENSES

	HUSBAND	WIFE	JOINT
Mortgage or rent			
Utilities			
Telephone			
Repairs			
Home maintenance			
Homemaker services			
Legal/Accounting			
Equipment rentals			
Insurance premiums			
Medicare			
Medigap			
Long-term care			
Disability			
Homeowners			
Life			
Automobile			
Other			
Personal care			
Food			
Clothing			
Auto/Transportation			
Medical/Dental (unreimbursed)			
Medication			

EXPENSES (Cont'd)

	HUSBAND	WIFE	JOINT
Payments			
Auto			
Credit cards			
Second home			
Other			
Gifts			
Entertainment			
Travel			
Charitable contributions			
Other long-term debt			
Federal taxes			
State/Local taxes			

STEP 12—COMPLETE A STATEMENT OF YEARLY INCOME AND EXPENSES

Every business prepares income and expense statements to see how it is doing. Your parents should do this also. Yearly income and expenses need to be matched for several reasons: to identify areas where expenses may be reduced or income increased; to explore ways to put income and expenses in better balance; and finally, to forecast increases in expenses and design both a timetable and a financial strategy for meeting them.

Approach the following list as you did the others. That is, pick out what applies and customize it.

Where will you find the information you need to complete this statement? Basic information on yearly income will come from your parents' past tax returns, year-end stock statements, and bank receipts. Paid checks and bills will provide raw data on expenses. If your parents pay bills with cash, ask them to save the receipts and record daily expenses in a notebook for a few weeks. If they pay by credit card this task is simpler, since each credit card company sends monthly statements. Some universal cards like American Express also produce year-end statements totaling detailed expenses by such categories as restaurants, hotels, transportation, and merchandise.

ANNUAL INCOME AND EXPENSE STATEMENT

_____

DATE

A. ANNUAL INCOME

	TAXABLE	NONTAXABLE
Wages, salaries		
Other compensation		
Interest		
Investment		
Rental or business income		
Social Security		
Pensions		
Annuity		
IRA/Keogh		
Rent		
Royalties		
Trust		
Other		

B. ANNUAL EXPENSES

	DEDUCTIBLE	NONDEDUCTIBLE
Mortgage or rent		
Utilities		
Telephone		
Repairs		

ANNUAL EXPENSES (CONT'D)

	DEDUCTIBLE	NONDEDUCTIBLE
Home maintenance		
Homemaker services		
Legal/Accounting		
Equipment rentals		
Insurance premiums		
Medicare		
Medigap		
Long-term care		
Disability		
Homeowners		
Life		
Automobile		
Other		
Personal care		
Food		
Clothing		
Auto/Transportation		
Medical/Dental (unreimbursed)		
Medication		
Payments		
Auto		
Credit cards		
Second home		
Gifts		

ANNUAL EXPENSES (CONT'D)

	DEDUCTIBLE	NONDEDUCTIBLE
Entertainment		
Travel		
Charitable contributions		
Other long-term debt		
Federal taxes		
State/Local taxes		

STEP 13—SIMPLIFY ROUTINE FINANCIAL TRANSACTIONS

Your parents can save time and aggravation by reducing the number of financial institutions they deal with and simplifying the way they pay bills, make deposits, or conduct other financial transactions. Here are a few suggestions:

- If tracking medical bills and insurance claims or balancing the checkbook is getting too complicated, seek help through a certified medical claims management service or similar services offered by your parents' local bank or a known bookkeeper.

- If transportation is a problem and safe deposit boxes, checking, money-fund, and savings accounts are scattered at different places, consolidate accounts at one location convenient to your parents' present home.

- Arrange for direct electronic deposit of Social Security benefits, civil service annuities, Veterans Administration payments, disability, pension, and Supplemental Security Income (SSI) checks into parents' financial accounts. This eliminates the delay and uncertainty of checks getting stolen, misplaced, destroyed, or lost in the mail. It also saves time in banking, and ensures a steady income stream when there is no one home to receive or deposit checks. To do this, your parents must complete Form SF 1199 (available at local bank branches) or call the Social Security Administration at 1-800-772-1213. If your parents anticipate a change in banks after this form is filed, notify Social Security immediately. It takes about three months to put direct deposit in place or make later changes.

· Whether your parents stash bonds or stock certificates in a safe deposit box or under their mattress, consider shifting these income-bearing certificates into an insured account in their name at a reputable brokerage house. This assures that subsequent coupon, dividend, and interest payments are automatically deposited into their account and can easily be used to meet your parents' changing financial needs. For example, by prior instruction to the broker, payments can be forwarded to an interest-bearing fund with check-writing privileges, used to purchase shares in another investment fund, or consolidated for monthly, quarterly, or semi-annual payments. Computers have made these financial instructions simple to execute and easy to alter.

A second advantage of shifting securities to a brokerage house comes if you should need to manage your parents' investments. Then you will find that securities held in a "street name" (the name of the brokerage house) instead of individual names can be sold more readily. For instance, if your parents cannot sign their papers and you are signing for them, stock transfer agents are sometimes reluctant to accept such "alternate signatures," even where state law authorizes this practice. With "street name" certificates, neither you nor your parents have to sign upon sale.

Step 14—Gain Access to Parents' Finances for Unexpected Situations

By now you have probably noticed how little access you have in an emergency. You already have begun to prepare for the unexpected by securing entry to your parents' safe deposit box through a signature card. Now work with them to grant you access to their financial accounts, should the need arise.

This may be a touchy subject. You may meet stiff resistance due to your parents' desire for privacy and total control over their money. But this step is very important. Explain that it lets you help out in minor accidents or emergencies—for example, if your widowed mother breaks her wrist and cannot write checks to cover her rent. Or if, while your parents are on vacation, a large insurance bill is due. Financial access in these circumstances makes life easier. Should parents become incapacitated, such access is an absolute necessity.

- Become an alternate signator to your parents' checking and savings accounts so you have emergency withdrawal and check-writing authority.

- Call their broker, insurance company, or other financial institutions to ask for appropriate power of attorney forms. Not all institutions will accept the form you might use. Some require you to use their language.

- Keep spare checks from each of these accounts in your own files.

Step 36 on p. 190 gives more details on the kind of legal authority you may need to gain access to your parents finances. Besides reducing hassles, these measures may avoid costly and complicated procedures if your parents need to go to a long-term care facility, cannot manage their own accounts, and leave you as the responsible party. If they do not want you to have this responsibility, encourage them to use the services of a lawyer or some other delegate they trust.

Step 15—Complete a Net Worth Statement

Retirement may lower your parents' income. But income alone does not reflect total wealth. For a complete picture you must also look behind the bills and receipts—at outstanding debt as well as home ownership, savings, and other assets. For example, the median annual income of families with heads of household ages sixty-five and over was $26,500 in 1994. For elderly persons not living in families, the median income was $11,500. Approximately 65 percent of both groups owned their own homes, with four-fifths living mortgage free, and over half owned a car, stock, bonds, or savings certificates and carried no debt.

A Net Worth Statement gives a snapshot of your parents' savings (assets) and debts (liabilities). When you subtract debts from savings you calculate "net worth." This statement should not take long to do, since the numbers will come from the financial documents you already have completed.

NET WORTH STATEMENT

_____

DATE

ASSETS   LIABILITIES

Cash   _____   Debts   _____

Cash surrender/Insurance   _____   Mortgage—home _____

Market value—Stocks/Bonds   _____   Mortgage—other _____

Deferred compensation   _____   Other debts   _____

IRAs   _____   Unpaid taxes   _____

Keoghs   _____

Annuity   _____

Market value—residence   _____

Market Value—other real estate_____

Loans receivable   _____

Cash value—business   _____

Cash value—automobiles   _____

Cash value—household items   _____

          Total assets _____   Total liabilities _____

Total assets _____ – Total liabilities _____   = Net worth _____

PLUGGING INTO THE NETWORKS

If you have concluded that it is time to step up to the plate and "do something" for your parents, one of the greatest possible favors is to find out what community resources and eldercare experts exist and how you and your parents can use them. You can do this before you have completed the previous steps.

Anyone who has traveled the eldercare road knows it is not unusual to face legal, insurance, housing, homecare, health, financial, transportation, medication, and emotional issues—simultaneously.

When such situations arise, "just-in-time access"—finding good, reliable information when you need it—is a must. And while it would be nice to place one call to learn all you need to know, the reality is that you must plug into multiple networks, hoping some of them will lead you down the right paths. You can ask a friend. You can ask the family doctor. You can talk to older neighbors. If you work for a large organization, you can meet its employee benefits staff. You can scan the telephone book. You can go to the library. Or you can go "online" (see p. 117).

Money, time, or lack of services—the normal roadblocks you might expect to encounter—are not the only issues. A fundamental obstacle to information lies in the words themselves. Because there is no standard "eldercare" vocabulary, there is no agreement even on what to call older people. The basic terms "Aging," "Senior" and "Elders" are Captain Marvel's "shazams" or Ali Baba's "abracadabras" to open many doors. But these keywords don't always work.

The result is that families shopping for eldercare support in telephone directories geared more to manufacturing than services often cannot locate the resources they seek. They do not know the proper terms or where to look. The "Blue Pages" of the White Pages are somewhat better for locating government services and information on government benefit programs. But there is little uniformity in terms describing similar for-profit and non-profit private services. For example, the Alzheimer's Association has over 250 chapters around the nation. But if your loved one is one of an estimated four million afflicted with the disease and you pick up a telephone directory to find help, you might look under the White Pages of the Yellow Pages, but not the Blue Pages of the White Pages, nor the Yellow Pages of the Yellow Pages, or even the Orange pages of either one. And there is no standard for the various books around the country.

This problem is compounded by the lack of common "headings" in Yellow-Page directories published by companies in different locations. For example, while there are listings for specific products such as "Artificial Eyes" or "Wheelchairs," directory advertising is not subdivided by specific topic such as social services, transportation, support groups, prosthetic devices, rehabilitative therapies, or housing alternatives.

Searching for "Senior Housing" means turning to "Adult Care Facilities" or "Residential Care Facilities" in the Southern New England Yellow Pages but "Assisted Living" in Georgia. In California, consumers can try "Congregate Living Health Facilities" (Pacific Bell), or, if you have a GTE book, "Adult Congregate Living Facilities" or perhaps "Homes-Domiciliary."

Small wonder our fingers have a hard time "walking" through the phone book when we try to help a relative cross-country. And this basic access problem holds just as true for library research, where we may discover terms cross-referenced under the archaic, now-unfamiliar, keyword "Aged."

What experienced caregivers have learned the hard way, and "information disseminators" are just figuring out, is that for the complex issues of eldercare *there is no single, direct-entry, standardized, nationwide integrated health and human services information system*. Only recently have human-service and information brokers made serious attempts to establish base definitions and common terminology. Only very recently have there been serious policy efforts at the national level to coordinate eldercare and disability lexicons and services.

The good news for caregivers of the elderly is that there *are* services available. Many of them. And there is a large network of information. Back in 1965, the same year Congress passed Medicare and Medicaid, it passed the Older Americans Act. That Act created a national network of public and private agencies which provides information about state and local senior citizen programs and caregiving services. All persons over sixty are eligible for services. No income tests are required to use these networks.

Under the 1965 Act, states distribute federal funds through the Area Agencies on Aging, which contract locally for various services provided to seniors and those who care for them. Presently 670 Area Agencies serve as focal points for aging services. They coordinate and fund more than 25,000 service-providing organizations throughout the country. Through these networks, seniors are served meals at community nutrition sites; delivered meals at home; or ride special transportation services to get to healthcare, medical screening, and leisure activities. More than $1.4 billion in federal funds alone was appropriated for such Older American Act Programs for 1995.

Your parents may already know about and use these senior programs. Or they may know about them but choose to ignore them because they are "just for old people." Nevertheless, you need to know they exist and how to find them. Here's how.

STEP 16—CALL YOUR LOCAL OFFICE ON AGING

They will help connect you to services in your parents' area. The National Eldercare Locator number (1-800-677-1116) can link you to your local office of the Area Agency on Aging. These offices are scattered about each state and serve all local counties. Using the Locator number is the most efficient way to reduce frustration when you begin your search, because these agencies are known by different names in different locales. Some have vague names like "Special Services Agency" or "Intergovernmental Council." Usually the term "Aging" or "Senior" or "Elder" appears somewhere in the name. If you cannot reach the Locator, and are calling long distance, have the operator search under "Division of Elder Affairs," "Area Agency on Aging," "Office on Aging," "Council on Aging," or "County Office on Aging."

Once you jump this hurdle, you will find some help. Whatever the labels, all these entities operate under the umbrella of State Departments of Aging and are fueled by federal, state, and local funds. They offer a wide range of professional social services, volunteer-based programs, and recreational/educational activities similar to items listed in the "Community Services" guide following this section.

For example, some local services available in Pennsylvania are: adult day-care centers, telephone reassurance, and chore services, transportation, employment, friendly visitor, and casework services. (Caseworkers help make arrangements to match special needs with special programs, help in managing personal and financial affairs, or offer assistance to seniors in risk of injury or abuse.) Other programs include Senior Centers which offer information, training, meals, and services to help place dependent adults in sheltered residential settings.

CONSUMER BEWARE

Calling the Eldercare Locator does not mean that all agencies referred are the same! Not only do the names of Area Agencies on Aging differ, their services vary as well. In fact, the "aging network" is more like a patchwork quilt. Local agencies differ widely in budget, scope, sophistication, and quality of service. Some agencies are terrific despite shrinking budgets. Others lack not only manpower and funding but a genuine mission. It is possible that your call will be answered by an answering machine, or busy signal. But don't give up. Remember, you can learn from every source.

STEP 17—USE PRECISE AND ASSERTIVE TELEPHONE TACTICS

While some consumers enjoy the challenge of telephone research, most of us freeze at the prospect of talking to strangers when we need help. This is especially true when we are unsure what kind of information we want. Here are some techniques to help you tackle the task:

- Before calling, have a pad of paper and a pencil handy. (A spiral notebook is better than loose-leaf paper, since it is harder to misplace.) With pad and pencil you can take notes during the conversation and record names, addresses, and phone numbers for later use.

- Be prepared to make at least seven calls before you find the information you want, and remind yourself to hang in there until you are confident you are on the right track. The more precisely you can identify your need, the faster you will get the right response.

- Be polite, be sympathetic, be charming, be grateful—but be firm. If the person on the other end of the line does not seem to understand your problem, ask to speak to a supervisor. Try not to lose your temper before you hang up, at least not on the first attempt. You can learn something from every call.

- Depending on which organizations or agencies you are calling, different methods of reaching them may be effective. If you are trying to reach a caseworker at a local Social Service agency, place your call early in the morning or right after lunch. In contrast, Social Security personnel recommend that if you need to call, and it is not an emergency, phone in the afternoon, and towards the end of the week or month to avoid getting a busy signal.

· Get the name and telephone number of everyone to whom you speak. If he or she can't help you, don't hang up until you obtain another name and number to call.

Finally, and most important of all:

•No matter who you call, be prepared to give specific information. Knowing precise details about the older person's health, functional status, and financial position helps cut red tape and lets others point you in the right direction faster. For example, "My mom's leg is in a cast, and she's using a wheelchair. She needs transportation to physical therapy twice a week. She is on Medicaid." You will get faster results stating that than the more general statement "I need to talk to someone about transportation for my mother."

STEP 18—LOCATE AN INFORMATION AND REFERRAL SERVICE OR CALL A HOTLINE

Let's expand upon this example. To learn about local public, private, or voluntary transportation options, you should contact a local Information & Referral Service through the Area Aging Agency. Or you can enter through a more general service door like the United Way.

Locating the Information & Referral Services or Hotlines (buzzword I & R) is not always simple. Once more, the problem is terminology. As acknowledged in a 1995 publication of the Association of Information & Referral Systems, "over

90% of the (American) population does not recognize the term." It elaborates on the problem:

> Why has information and referral been an almost hidden part of the human services? It is largely because the services go under so many different names: FIRST CALL FOR HELP; COMMUNITY INFORMATION SERVICE; HELP LINE; IN-FORMATION AND ASSISTANCE; RESOURCE AND RE-FERRAL; THE (BLANK) HOT LINE and dozens more. There has never been a single, standard, identifying element in the names that would mark them as the same kinds of service." (Out of the Shadows—INFORMATION & REFERRAL: Bringing People and Services Together)

If you are calling long distance, don't give up. Within the last few years new crosswalks have emerged to connect long-distance caregivers with far away service providers.

For example, toll-free telephone *hotlines* provide I & R, literature, and other services. The Eldercare Locator Service (1-800-677-1116) (Monday–Friday 9 A.M.–11 P.M. est.) which helps people living far away find needed state or local information in the communities where their parents live is one example. ABLEDATA is another; this electronic database provides product information on 20,000 assistive devices for the handicapped and disabled from 3,000 manufacturers (1-800-346-2742). The National Health Information Center (1-800-336-4797) is a third. It offers I & R to groups, professional societies, and government agencies, as well as publications relating to health issues. Finally, the Visiting Nurse Association (1-800-426-2547) provides referrals to local nursing associations.

And there's more. Other national networks exist both in

the non-profit and for-profit sectors. One example is the Elder Support Network, a service for some 145 non-profit Jewish Family and Children's Agencies around the country.

At the workplace, a growing number of companies and government employers are contracting with private resource and referral services to meet the eldercare needs of their employees and retirees. Serving working members of the "sandwich generation," these companies began by providing help with childcare services and expanded their range to include eldercare. The Partnership Group in Blue Bell, Pennsylvania for example serves more than 150 mid- to large-size companies nationwide, with almost one million employees, retirees, and family members.

For a distraught employee trying to balance work and family issues, eldercare help is on the other end of a telephone line. Trained telephone consultants (with masters-level degrees) function as case managers to work with individual callers to develop "service plans" to meet each caller's specific needs. Issues range from living wills to housing alternatives. Written materials supplement the "high-touch" referral process. The Partnership referral network spans the country. So it can benefit the long-distance caregiver as well as the one across the street from mom and dad. Ask the human resource or benefits office of your employer to learn if your company sponsors such a service.

STEP 19—SEEK ADVICE FROM EXPERTS

The lists of Personal Documents, Medical History, the Personal Support System, and Financial Resources and Obligations you prepared in the last section provide the crucial data

National Eldercare Locator (1-800-677-1116)

ABLEDATA—assistive devices for the handicapped (1-800-346-2742)
National Health Information Center (1-800-336-4797)
Visiting Nurse Association (1-800-426-2547)
Alzheimer's Disease Education and Referral Center (ADEAR) (1-800-438-4380)

for professionals to incorporate in their assessments and recommendations when you seek expert advice.

If you feel a parent is at risk because of increasing mental confusion, or frailty, or forgetfulness, it may be both necessary and helpful to go outside individual-care channels for a full-scale evaluation and plan of action. Start with the family doctor. Ask where to go for a comprehensive geriatric assessment. The purpose of this review is to determine individual and family resources and strengths as well as problems.

A geriatric assessment is a formal review which includes the family, the individual, and an examination of medical records, as well as a complete physical and multidisciplinary evaluation. Assessment teams are generally located at private or public clinics and medical centers. The team consists of geriatric social workers, psychiatrists, geriatric medical specialists, and related healthcare professionals such as physical therapists or disease-specific counselors.

This assessment usually takes a few visits on an outpatient basis. Questions will focus on day-to-day functioning. The formal names of these gauges of functional capability are Activities of Daily Living and Instrumental Activities of Daily Living, also known as ADLs and IADLs. (ADLs include eating, dressing, bathing, taking medications, or going to the bathroom. IADLs include other home-managed activities, such as preparing meals, shopping, managing money, looking up telephone numbers, using the telephone, and doing laundry or other light housework.)

Your situation may not be so extreme, in which case, other levels of support are available. When planning long-term care options and costs, you and your parents will want to explore the suggestions offered by eldercare experts, certified accountants, lawyers, and investment or financial planners. For example,

- a social worker from the local Area Agency on Aging can offer advice on the availability of various community-supported benefits;

- a geriatric care manager may recommend home-based options, or refer you to a local adult day program:

- a financial planner might help you understand and coordinate all available medical, disability, and life insurance benefits and suggest reallocating savings from parents' passbook accounts, Treasury notes, or certificates of deposit into top-rated mutual fund portfolios of stocks and bonds paying higher dividends and having greater inflation protection;

- an insurance broker or pension advisor might recommend better ways to utilize your parents pension, borrowing against paid life insurance, IRA, and pension funds, or selling unneeded personal property to increase available cash reserves;

- a lawyer will help establish all necessary estate documents for asset protection and distribution and work on the details should they consider the option of equity-based financing on their home if they are "house rich" but "cash poor."

Of course you must check the reputation and reliability of any advisors before leaping to follow their suggestions. And remember to call an accountant for ways to minimize the tax bite of any financial recommendation.

STEP 20—JOIN A "SELF-HELP" SUPPORT GROUP

Private and non-profit networks help fill gaps in eldercare information and service. And what they do not offer, consumers can often supplement on their own by joining "self-help" support groups. (See p. 80 to learn more about other community resources, organizations, and agencies which may be useful in helping you make arrangements for your parents' care, now or in the future.)

These organizations provide an invaluable service in helping families cope. According to Ed Madara, Director of the American Self-Help Clearinghouse, such groups are valuable because of their basic characteristics: They provide mutual help, in which knowledge is pooled, experiences shared. They are composed of peers. They are voluntary and run by and for their members.

Thousands of self-help groups dot the country. They are sponsored by organizations including the Alzheimer's, Parkinson's, Arthritis, Cancer, and Stroke Associations, or by family caregiver organizations like Children of Aging Parents (CAPS) or the National Alliance for the Mentally Ill (NAMI). They may have offshoots in hospitals, nursing homes, and community centers, or they may have their own building. They do a solid job of providing practical information, resource materials, and honest appraisals of local services.

To find these groups, you can look up a particular organization in the White Pages of the telephone book, or, check Appendix 1 at the back of the book for local clearinghouse information. Then call for information, and attend a meeting. Even if your parent will not go, you will greatly benefit. (See Part Two—Gathering Resources, Section Two: Accessing Eldercare on the Information Highway p. 103 for more information about online support groups.)

Step 21—Obtain Directories of Information and Services and Review their Contents

Most I & R Services can tell you how to obtain a community resource guide for older adults, if one is available. Since directories are constantly changing as material is updated—and new groups and services emerge while old ones go out of business—you will want to keep a current directory handy. Just as there is an aging network, and an information and referral network, there is also a health network. Helpful information sharers can plug you into all three.

The following Community Resources Guide in Section One on pp. 77–99 offers a sample of eldercare community-based services, in-home services, and access services that may be available.

And, if you have access to the Internet, using resources identified in Section Two: Information and Resources on the Internet, as well as the Search Keyword Index (p. 265) at the end of the book may help you locate additional support.

PART TWO

GATHERING
RESOURCES

A COMMUNITY RESOURCES GUIDE

SECTION 1   A COMMUNITY RESOURCES GUIDE SUMMARY

I & R Services

· Adult/Continuing
    Education

· Adult Day Care

· Advocacy Organizations

· Caregiver Support

· Caregiver Training

· Care Management

· Chore Services

· Companionship Programs

· Consumer Help Services

· Counseling Services

· Delivery Services

· Emergency Services

· Employment

· Escort Services

· Financial Aid

· Foster Care/Residential
    Facilities

· Friendly Visiting

· Geriatric Assessment

· Health Information and
    Services

· Home-Delivered Meals

· Home Healthcare

· Home Improvement
    Services

· Homemaker Services

· Hospices

· Informal Support Systems

· Legal Services and
    Ombudsman Programs

· Library Programs

- Medication Management
- Mental Health Services
- Money Management Services
- Moving Services
- Nursing Home Ombudsmen
- Nutrition Services
- Personal Care (companion/caretaker)
- Recreation/Fitness/ Wellness Programs
- Respite Care
- Self-Help Programs
- Senior Centers
- Social Service Agencies
- Telephone Reassurance
- Transportation Services
- Volunteer Services

In an information age where too much data is overwhelming, and too little data, incapacitating, information specialists who help filter the useful from the useless are indispensable. They can save you time, energy, and expense. Eldercare Information and Referral Services (I & Rs) are available. Their staff should help you track down needed support and services. They provide information on community social services, such as consumer protection, home health, energy assistance, housing, legal assistance, and tax help. They also refer callers to appropriate resources which may provide these services. In addition, some may provide crisis counseling and problem solving on the telephone. Your first call should be to the Area Agency on Aging to get the number of the I & R Service in your parents area. To locate the Area Agency, call the Eldercare Locator number (1-800-677-1116) or check the telephone book under headings for "Aging," "Human Services Organizations" or "Senior" in the "Community Services" section of the White Pages or Blue Pages.

· *Adult/Continuing Education*—Local colleges, libraries, community centers, and museums may offer stimulating full-time, part-time, day, or evening programs and study tours for students of all ages. Local schools, community colleges, newspapers, magazines—even the local library—may stock course guides or brochures on available programs. Some programs may be free. Others may offer discounts for seniors. Retirement can offer your parent an opportunity to go back to school to pick up that college degree begun forty years earlier. It may also provide time to attend noncredit classes or hands-on programs of specific interest.

· *Adult Day Care*—This generally means a planned program of social and recreational activities, health services, and therapeutic activities provided in a safe nonresidential setting to persons who are not physically or mentally capable of being left alone. In 1994 an estimated 3,000 adult day-care centers operated as private non-profit entities. Many are located in hospitals, nursing homes, religious centers, or civic associations. Many are also sponsored by local governments. Most centers operate programs Monday–Friday and offer transportation as part of a daily fee. Fees can reach $60 per day, but are often set on a sliding scale, based on ability to pay. Some costs may be covered by Medicare, Medicaid, or certain long-term care insurance policies.

· *Advocacy Organizations*—These groups offer services and benefits which support volunteer work—as well as representation before government agencies—on special issues facing seniors. Such groups as the American Asso-

ciation of Retired Persons (AARP) (phone: 1-800-424-
2277), the Gray Panthers (phone: 202-387-3111), and the
Older Women's League (OWL) (phone: 202-783-6686)
have chapters all around the country. Check the White
Pages of the phone book to find a local chapter or call the
numbers above.

• *Caregiver Support* (see also Self-Help)—These self-help
groups may focus on broad topics such as medical assistance
or emotional loss or narrower topics, such as support in
dealing with specific conditions. Groups that relate to specific health problems such as care of Alzheimer's, heart disease, or cancer patients often have hundreds or thousands
of local units. For example, the Alzheimer's Association has
over 200 chapters nationwide which include more than
1,600 support groups. Self-help groups range from those
concerned with specific health issues to aid to individuals
coping with addictions, bereavement, disabilities, or mental health problems. The eldercare self-help groups share
information and provide emotional support and tips on
aging, being a caregiver, and related family issues. Some
national organizations you should know about are Children
of Aging Parents (CAPS) of Levittown, Pennsylvania
(phone: 1-800-227-7294) and the Well Spouse Foundation
of New York City (phone: 1-800-838-0879).

Many states also have self-help clearinghouses which
provide information and referral on all in-state self-help
groups. To find a group, check Appendix 1 or look for
"caregiver" or "self-help" in the health guides of the local
newspaper. Check for the name of the specific group in
the White Pages, or call a physician or local hospital.

• *Caregiving Training*—These programs educate caregivers in the basic information and techniques needed to effectively provide care to the elderly. To locate training programs, call the Red Cross, local hospitals, or Cooperative Extension Services. Ask about available courses, video, or print materials.

• *Care Management*—These agencies provide a full range of services for seniors, including assessments and care plans. They help connect older people with services they need so they can remain in the community with as much independence as possible. Public and private agencies such as the Community Alternative Systems Agency in New York, can assess parents' medical and social needs, perform detailed evaluations, develop care plans, provide counseling, and assign staff members (known as case managers) to coordinate and monitor care. For example, when a parent's day companion doesn't show up, or special coordination services are needed, the care manager can handle the problem so you don't get a panicked call when you've just arrived at work.

The local branch of the National Association of Social Workers (NASW) or parallel organizations can refer you to local social workers who specialize in such coordinated care. Private geriatric care managers have set up fee-for-service consulting businesses to act as proxies for adult children who live far from their parents. They can provide information on accessing public benefits, find suitable housing, coordinate home care and transportation services, monitor care, and handle emergencies. The National Association of Geriatric Care Managers (Tucson,

Arizona) publishes an annual directory of members located around the country.

· *Chore Services* (see separate list for Home Improvement Services)—These entities provide care of the home in such areas as cleaning, laundry, cooking, and shopping when parents cannot handle those tasks. In some states chore services also include minor home repairs, heavy housecleaning, and yard work. Chore services may be available alone or in combination with home health services. Your minister may know of volunteer services. To locate others, call a social service agency or Area Agency on Aging or check the Yellow Pages for "Housecleaning," "Home Maintenance," or "Home Health Services".

· *Companionship Programs* (see also Friendly Visiting and Telephone Reassurance and Respite Programs)—These are offered by many AARP chapters (phone: 1-800-424-2277), churches, and senior centers. Special widowed persons support groups and bereavement counseling are also available.

· *Consumer Help Services*—These services by individuals or agencies provide information services on various issues from credit counseling to legal action. For example, United Seniors Health Cooperative, a regional non-profit membership organization based in Washington D.C., offers timely publications and special reports on healthcare, housing, health insurance, and Medicaid.

The Better Business Bureau and various offices of Consumer Protection or Consumer Product Safety deal with consumer complaints and issues of consumer fraud. A local radio station or newspaper may also have a "Call for

Action" service for consumer complaints. They can be found in the phone book under Consumer Protection.

· *Counseling Services* (see separate section on Mental Health Services)—In your parents community the leading organization on aging will coordinate comprehensive services from housing to nutrition. For disease-specific issues, check the White Pages of the telephone book by the name of the condition or use the Eldercare Locator to identify specific issues such as housing or grief and loss counseling. You can also search under "Counseling—Personal and Family," "Clergy," "Clinics," "Marriage, Family, Child, and Individual Counselors," "Psychologists," "Social Service Organizations," and "Mental Health Services."

· *Delivery Services*—Many food markets, pharmacies, dry cleaners, video rental, department stores, and even cable TV offer shop-at-home or free home delivery services. You can also arrange for someone to do your parents' marketing, banking, and errands. Separate shopping services charge for that service. But for the homebound it's a lift to know that supermarkets—not to mention beauticians and barbers—can provide their services on the spot.

· *Emergency Services*—These range from crisis intervention hotlines through rescue squads to emergency numbers for gas and electric company power outages and leaks. Other emergency services include protective services to investigate reports of neglect, abuse, and exploitation of senior citizens; services to furnish food, clothing, supplies, or financial aid; and temporary shelters for those seeking emergency assistance. To locate services call 911.

In addition, Personal Emergency Response Systems

(PERS) can provide automatic responses to theft, fire, medical, or other emergencies through electronic monitors and backups. Activating an attachment on the telephone or a device worn on the person will alert local police or rescue squads in the event of emergency. There is usually a modest monthly fee for this service. Monitoring systems can be found in the Yellow Pages under "Medical Alarms" or "Security Systems."

· *Employment*—While life expectancy is increasing, for many older workers, corporate and government downsizing, mechanization, and global competition have limited the length of their careers. Yet earning income beyond formal retirement is a necessity for many whose watches may tick on their wrists for thirty more years. Older workers have new training opportunities and need to tap into programs that help them find and retain jobs. Organizations like the AARP, the Jewish Council for the Aging, the National Council on Aging, and the National Caucus and Center on Black Aged may have an employment program in your parents' community. Check the local Office on Aging and the local division of employment services, as well.

· *Escort Services*—These people accompany those too frail to go out alone to shop, go to the doctor, or anywhere else. Both volunteer and paid escort services are available through social service agencies or many religious institutions.

· *Financial Aid*—Various local or federal government and charitable benefit programs exist to help those in need.

To find them, check the Information and Referral Services under "Community Information," "Helpline," "Senior Information," "United Way," and, if relevant, the Social Security Administration and the Veterans Administration.

· *Foster Care / Residential Facility*—These services help place an eligible individual who needs care in a single-family home which agrees to provide meals, housekeeping, and personal care. Expenses are paid to the host family from public funds. Contact a central referral bureau, a church-based group like Catholic Charities, or a local government human service or aging agency for details.

· *Friendly Visiting*—This service provides volunteers from churches, synagogues, or social agencies who visit the homebound to provide companionship and neighborly services such as writing letters, running errands—or just listening. A call to a local agency on aging, the AARP, or your parent's minister will guide you to volunteer groups to contact.

· *Geriatric Assessment*—This is a comprehensive evaluation of parent's mental, physical, and social condition conducted with parent and family members by a professional team at private or public clinics and medical centers. The team makes recommendations to the older person—as well as that person's family and his or her primary care physician—on medical, social, and financial options (see p. 70).

· *Health Information and Services*—These range from information on where to get help in completing medical claims forms, to services that help resolve medical bill problems or provide counseling on health insurance.

They include multiservice organizations like the Red Cross and many university medical centers as well as programs sponsored by the Visiting Nurse Association and public libraries. For example, the Regional Library in Wheaton, Maryland has a Health Information Center which covers topics such as medications, stress, mental health, nursing homes, and allergies. Readers have access to a special subject guide and computerized databases. Librarians can search specialized medical databases for more information.

In addition to the resources listed online (see pp. 121–36), there are self-help groups for just about every medical condition identified. Some examples are the Arthritis Foundation, American Cancer Society, Self-Help for Hard of Hearing People (SHHH), Columbia Lighthouse for the Blind, and the American Heart Association. For a listing of national organizations, locate a copy of *The Self-Help Sourcebook* published by the American Self-Help Clearinghouse in Denville, New Jersey (1-201-625-9565) or check the resource section of former First Lady Rosalynn Carter's excellent caregiver's book, *Helping Yourself Help Others* (see Appendix 3).

• *Home-Delivered Meals*—Meals on Wheels, a volunteer private-sector program, provides one hot meal and a light supper once each day, five days a week to the homebound. Weekend or seven-day delivery is available in some locations. Participants pay for the cost of the meal, but free delivery is a community service furnished by volunteers. Fees vary. Subsidized delivery may also be available through the Area Agency on Aging. Look in the Business Listings of the Yellow Pages for the local program. In 1993 nearly 106 million home-delivered meals were served to 825,000 disabled homebound elders. Meals on Wheels programs are listed in the White Pages of the telephone book. Many restaurants and private caterers also offer meal-delivery services. They are listed under "Caterers" in the Yellow Pages.

· *Home Healthcare* (see Homemaker Services)—This includes a wide range of services from nursing care, physical therapy, hearing care, occupational or speech therapy, nutrition, counseling by a social worker, and home-maker/health aides. Often services are coordinated through a home healthcare agency led by a nurse operating under physician's orders. Fees vary with type of agency and length and types of service. Special home care groups also support the efforts of families coping with Alzheimer's disease.

If your parent is coming home from the hospital and needs special care that you cannot provide, a social worker known as a "hospital discharge planner" should help you design a care plan to maximize care with available resources. While designing this plan, find out what services will be covered under Medicare, Medicaid, or private insurance, and for how long. Some hospitals provide direct in-home health services for their discharged patients. To find help, start by gathering referrals from the inner circle of parent's relatives, neighbors, and friends. Then call the local Visiting Nurse Association or Area Agency on Aging, or check classified directories under "Home Health Services" (see p. 210).

· *Home Improvement Services*—Some local governments help low-income seniors with home improvement and disability modifications. Religious institutions and high schools with community service programs also organize periodic campaigns of volunteers who undertake free projects to repair or modify the homes of low-income seniors and the disabled. One national program called "Christmas in April" sends volunteer workers free of charge on the last Saturday and/or Sunday in April. As with other community services, call the local Area Agency on Aging for Information and Referral on specific programs.

In the community you may also find businesses like the Home Connections Referral Service of Silver Spring, Maryland, which offer phone advice on home maintenance, cleaning, repair, and improvements. Callers ask about approved firms that service their neighborhood. Approved firms are screened for reliability and quality.

ABLEDATA, the National Rehabilitation Information Center in Washington, D.C., has a toll-free number (1-800-346-2742) which provides information for people seeking assistive equipment, devices, and furniture to help the disabled. An information specialist can help match product to need.

· *Homemaker Services* (see also Personal Care)—Homemaker aides carry out light housekeeping and household management tasks. They also can assist your parent with walk-

ing, bathing, dressing, eating, errands, and escorts. Sometimes, under supervision, they administer medications
and make progress reports. These services are not considered skilled services. They are not covered by Medicare.
However, if your parent is collecting SSI, is aged, blind, or
disabled, they *may* be covered under Medicaid, the VA, or
other in-home state support programs. To locate them,
check community service agencies and directories under
"Home Health Care" or "Homemaker-Home Health Aide."
The classified section of the Sunday newspaper might also
bring just the right person into your lives. Naturally, this
last route may involve more time spent on reference
checking and training (see also Step 40, p. 210).

· *Hospices*—These offer supportive programs for the care of
terminally ill patients and their families either at home or
in special skilled-care facilities. Their emphasis is on pain
control, symptom management, and family counseling.
The hospice mission is generally to treat the physical,
emotional, and spiritual needs of the patient. For more information, call the National Hospice Helpline (1-800-
658-8898).

· *Informal Support Systems*—Don't forget your friends,
parents' friends, and the informal support networks of
neighbors, cousins, godchildren, or lifelong advisors and
caregivers on whom you and they have always relied (see
p. 34).

· *Legal Services and Ombudsmen Programs*—(See also Nursing
Home Ombudsmen). The Lawyer Referral and Information Service of the local bar association is a good place to
begin. Some local law schools have special advocacy pro-

grams for seniors. Federal agencies such as the Legal Services Corporation or chapters of national organizations
such as the Legal Counsel for the Elderly of the AARP provide legal services to those who need assistance with public benefits, wills, taxes, Social Security, Medicare claims,
Medicaid coverage, SSI, disability, litigation, and protective services. Check the telephone directory or call the
local AARP chapter for further information.

You don't have to pay a lot of money for basic legal information and documents. Families looking for information on advance directives can call the local medical or
hospital association or the AARP to receive a copy of a
healthcare decision-making guide combining the living
will and healthcare power of attorney (see Step 36). Send
your request and $2.00 for the booklet *Shape Your Health
Care Future with Health Care Advance Directives* (D15803) to
AARP Fulfillment (EE0940), 601 E St. NW, Washington,
D.C. 20049. The local stationery store may also sell basic
standardized forms valid in the state where your parents
live.

· *Library Programs*—Along with resource centers and skilled
librarians who can help you or your parents search for information in the library or through the Internet, libraries
provide numerous outreach programs (see p. 86). Book-
mobiles may service senior living sites. The homebound
can be supplied with books and video tapes monthly. If
your parents have visual handicaps, the Library of Congress offers large print and "talking books" delivered or
mailed to individuals' homes (write to National Library

Service for the Blind and Physically Handicapped, Washington, DC 20542; or call 1-800-424-8567). Private companies offer mail-order rentals of audio books. The National Association of Radio Reading Services provides the handicapped access to information from print by distributing a free special radio receiver through the local reading service. Call the NARRS office at 412-488-3944 for a referral. If parents have a hearing problem, librarians can also tell you how to gain access to teletype machines which allow deaf people to place telephone calls.

· *Medication Management*—According to a 1995 GAO report, nearly five million elderly Americans take prescription drugs that are unsuitable or outdated and can lead to "medical crises resulting in hospitalization or death." "Adverse Reactions," "Contraindications," and "Effectiveness" are all words you should ask your pharmacist and physician about to make sure your elderly family member is not one of these millions. While you are at the drug store, ask about seven-day pill reminder containers and easy-open medicine bottles. Ask the doctor and pharmacist about side effects of nonprescription drugs and vitamin supplements. The local pharmacist is an invaluable resource. Often he is the only one with enough information to identify bad interactions or adverse drug-related symptoms. (See Step 37, p. 198 for more questions to ask about new medications.)

· *Mental Health Services*—An estimated 15 percent of older people suffer from mental health problems, such as depression, which affect how they care for themselves. Depression can easily be caused by the losses, physical impairments, and health changes affecting an older person. The good news is that depression can be treated successfully more than 75 percent of the time. Many support services are available to help. They include diagnostic assessment, crisis intervention, medication management, individual counseling, and psychotherapy (both for substance abuse problems and/or mental illness), as well as day treatment programs and outpatient clinics. Individual, family, or group therapy programs may be based in hospitals or in community settings. Talk with your own doctor as well as your parents for referrals and assistance. The strain of caregiving often leads to depression for caregivers as well as those whose needs they are attending.

• *Money Management Services*—Accountants, banks, trained volunteers from the AARP, and private businesses are all available to help manage finances. Many of these charge a fee, but many offer services on a sliding scale based on ability to pay. Their services now include balancing checkbooks, paying bills, organizing records, establishing budgets, and settling problems with creditors.

Sometimes these services also help gather records for income tax preparation. If you or a trusted friend have power of attorney for a loved one, you will want to coordinate money management with other tasks such as medical insurance filing and investment review. If you are the one helping, a home computer software program such as *Quicken* may help simplify these tasks. If there is no one to help, call the AARP or Social Security Administration and ask about the "Representative Payee Project," a voluntary service for older people who can no longer manage their financial affairs.

· *Moving Services*—These are provided by "relocation consultants" who can do everything from helping your family organize for a parents' move to planning for the sale of property, through disposing of unwanted household items, arranging for cleaning of the old home, or coordinating the move and unpacking at the other end. Since this is a stressful time for families, particularly for a parent who has been settled in one location for many years, you may find that a third party can do a much better job than you in helping organize the move to a new place. They can help you find the outlets to sell or dispose of unwanted possessions. They may charge by the hour or take a percentage of collected funds. Having an estate sale, or selling through auction houses, consignment shops, or antique dealers, can turn unwanted items into needed cash. And charitable organizations always need clothing, bedding, books, and home products. Real estate agents are valuable sources of referral information and assistance for these services (see Step 41, p. 215).

· *Nursing Home Ombudsmen*—These positions are funded and mandated by federal law. Ombudsmen are trained volunteers who monitor the quality of life for residents in nursing homes. They act as the residents' advocate in resolving complaints. Call the Area Agency on Aging or inquire at the nursing home, which is required to give residents and families the name and telephone number of the local ombudsman.

• *Nutrition Services*—According to background materials from the 1995 White House Conference on Aging, nutrition-related conditions affect 85 percent of the elderly and contribute significantly to needless hospitalizations. Food-related problems are a big issue for people living alone, but there are also many services available to help address them. For example, in 1993 the Older Americans Act funded nearly 135 million meals provided to 2.5 million seniors in communal settings such as senior centers, housing projects, churches, synagogues, and schools. Social activities, health screening, exercise, and information and recreation programs are important additions to these communal meals. The meal is free, but participants are invited to contribute as they can to cover its cost. Some communities sponsor public/private partnerships which provide for weekend services when communal or Meals on Wheels services are generally unavailable.

• *Personal Care (companion/caretaker)*—This is another buzzword for custodial in-home care to help with feeding, toileting, dressing, bathing, combing hair, and trimming nails of older people. As you may have noticed, there is a confusing overlap of terminology between Personal Care, Homemaker, Chore Service, and Health Aide services. When requesting aid, families should specify the *tasks* needed to be done, not the type of worker. Families should also check under "Senior Citizens Service Organizations." While Medicare generally does not pay for these services, they are considered "dependent care" deductions when filing tax returns. If a parent is disabled and eligible for Medicaid, these services may be covered (see Step 33, p. 168).

· *Recreation / Fitness / Wellness Programs*—A major growth industry in the past decade, line dancing, chair exercises, Tai Chi, square dancing, walking clubs, dance exercise programs, Yoga, stretching, weight-lifting, and aqua-aerobics for the fit and arthritic alike are found all across the country. Many health clubs offer special discounts for seniors using daytime hours. Community centers, recreation departments, physical therapy centers, senior centers, "Ys," and local senior associations are all good sources of information on program start dates or continuing courses. Suburban apartment buildings with large senior populations may offer "in-house" programs. Should your parent prefer the privacy of a bedroom for "setting up" routines, you can rent or purchase videotapes for any fitness level. Once you start looking, you will find programs everywhere.

· *Respite Care*—is an aging network term. It refers to hours or several days of temporary relief designed to aid primary family caregivers. These assistance services are organized by churches and synagogues, hospices, nursing homes, assisted-living facilities, home health agencies, and volunteer agencies. It is always a good idea to schedule well in advance of need. To find out about costs and availability of respite care in your parent's area, check their local directory of aging services, or call a self-help group like the Alzheimer's Association.

- *Self-Help Programs*—From managing breast cancer to living with Alzheimer's disease, consumers over the past two decades have learned to be more active and informed in improving their own health and choosing appropriate services. Countering and gradually changing a professional climate that traditionally served to limit consumer or patient access to information and restrict individual's ability to make informed choices, self-help groups have become an increasingly valuable access route to resources as well as providing a needed forum for sharing good and bad experiences (see Step 20, p. 73). Some groups servicing older adults are Grandparents Raising Grandchildren, Forty Plus (a job-search support group for unemployed managers, executives, and professionals), and the Widowed Persons Service of the AARP.

- *Senior Centers*—Senior centers are part of the Aging Network. They offer a variety of social, health, nutritional, educational, and recreational services. Many provide transportation from home to their activities. In addition to serving as meeting places, they often offer counseling, group meals, special trips, legal services, and financial advice. Call the local Area Agency on Aging Information and Referral Service to locate centers in your area. Ask about programs and transportation as well.

- *Social Service Agencies*—Government, community non-profit, religious, family service, and hospital-based programs for the elderly include adult day care, I & R, transportation, in-home care, and volunteer opportunities. Specific agencies also offer assessments, escort transportation, and homemaker services. Other agencies

handle cases involving older adults who are abused or ne-
glected or need crisis care or family support. Again, call
the Eldercare Locator, or local I & R, for a referral to the
agency in your parents' area.

· *Telephone Reassurance*—A volunteer makes daily telephone
calls at prearranged times to elderly persons living alone
to see if all is well. If the person does not answer, neighbors or police are alerted. Churches, synagogues, or Visiting Nurse Associations often provide these services. If
your parent has a weak support structure of family and
friends, the local Area Agency on Aging I & R is a gateway
to this valuable service.

· *Transportation Services*—By law, transportation support for
older people is a covered benefit incorporated in certain
federal statutes. For example, Medicare and Medicaid may
cover stretcher service to the hospital and some outpatient
hospital procedures. When seeking assistance with transportation, it is important to specify parents' functional
level of ability. For example, "curb to curb" transport services require that the rider be able to walk from house to
curb to enter a vehicle. "Door to Door" services assist or
carry passengers who cannot walk from their home to the
vehicle.

It is also important to identify the purpose of travel and
its degree of urgency. For example, there are distinctions
between emergency and nonemergency medical transport. You may need a rescue squad or ambulance service
during an emergency. Or perhaps your parent only needs
transport for individually scheduled trips to a physician's
office, medical clinic, hospital, or other medical facility;

a less rapid and less expensive bus, van, or taxi may be appropriate.

Nonmedical transport includes shared-ride systems for shopping, socializing, recreation, group meals, and visits to social service organizations. To find these systems, first ask around. Then check classified directories under "Disability Services" and "Handicapped Transportation." These categories should cross reference to other sections such as "Ambulance Service," "Buses—Charter and Rental," and "Taxicab."

For example, the 1995 *Resource Guide* published by Iona Senior Services in Washington, D.C. (phone: 202-966-1055) lists four types of transportation for a "variety of essential needs" arranged through public, for-profit, and voluntary organizations. Information on public transportation includes telephone numbers for bus routes, how to get reduced fares for seniors, handicapped access information, and how to make reservations to ride lift-equipped buses for the handicapped (called "kneeling buses"). The *Greater Cincinnati Older Adult Resource Guide* (phone: 513-871-4737) offers information on hospitals providing nonmedical transport as well as independent senior centers and community transportation resources. One example is a service in which volunteers drive members to medical appointments, shopping, and banking visits in their own cars.

· *Volunteer Services*—Many services listed above rely on volunteer help. Adult day care, friendly visiting, home care support, intergenerational programs, escorts, ombudsmen, nutrition programs, medical claims assistance, recreation, and telephone reassurance programs are staffed by volunteers. The Retired Senior Volunteer Program (RSVP) and the Senior Corps of Retired Executives (SCORE) are federal programs worth learning more about. The telephone numbers of local programs are listed in the White Pages of the telephone book.

ACCESSING ELDERCARE ON THE INFORMATION HIGHWAY

A good friend of mine recently found out that both her mother and her father had been told they have cancer. She visited me one evening. It was the lack of information that was her first frustration, she said. Her parents were too afraid to ask the doctors much, and my friend was too afraid to ask her parents much.

We got on the Web and entered "cancer" as a search command. Nearly a thousand entries popped up. Click here and we could go to Onco Link or Cancer Net or the National Cancer Institute's databases. Click here . . . and we could read about new treatments. Click here and we could read stories of other people losing parents to cancer. My friend did a lot of clicking and downloading, then she did a lot of reading.

And then she began talking to her parents. And they all began talking to the doctors. The three of them don't know yet how things will turn out, but now they're facing fate as a family.

How strange to think that all this power is just sitting up there waiting to be pulled down, as if from the clouds. *

*Jeanne Marie Laskas, "The Power and the Glory," *Washington Post Magazine*, April 23, 1995.

Fast, low-cost electronic technology can dramatically expand the abilities of families, service providers, and employers to conveniently find resources and practical measures that improve the care and well-being of America's elderly. This powerful new weapon belongs in all consumers' eldercare tool kits. It allows families to overcome frustrating obstacles to effective decision making. Those obstacles include the invisibility of needed services; limited exchange of information; poor search or navigation tools; and weak connections between current "stand-alone" information systems.

The "information highway" helps to overcome these barriers.

If you are already familiar with this road, skip this introductory section and instead go directly to either "Eldercare: Possibilities and Pitfalls" (see page 117), or Section 3: A Sampler of Eldercare Internet Addresses starting on page 121. If not, you may find the following short tour helpful.

WELCOME TO CYBERSPACE

Time magazine has described the Internet as a "vast international network of networks that enables computers of all kinds to share services and communicate directly, as if they were part of one giant, seamless, global computing machine." The Net links commercial online services like America Online and CompuServe with over 50,000 university, corporate, and government computer networks.

Step 22—Learn the Primary Roads, Symbols, and Signposts of the Information Highway

The information highway is divided between communication and resources. Using an Internet address a user can send and receive mail electronically. Using a *Uniform Resource Locator* (URL), a user can locate Internet sites, review what they contain, and transfer information to a personal computer.

· *Internet Address*—Each part of an Internet address used for communication means something. The address is typed in lower case letters without any spaces. The first part of the address tells "who" the user is. The @ ("at") symbol separates the "who" from the "where," the location and domain of the user's server computer. (This is the name of the computer that connects to the Internet community.) The name and status of the location are usually three-letter suffixes, set apart by a period. Here are the common suffixes:

> .com (commercial)
> .edu (educational)
> .gov (government)
> .mil (military)
> .net (networking)
> .org (noncommercial)

If you wanted to send me an electronic letter, and I subscribed to a commercial service like America Online, my Internet address would be njlevin@aol.com.

· *Uniform Resource Locator (URL)*—Unlike Internet addresses for communication, the URL is the address for a source of concentrated information. The URL address contains four parts: the protocol type, the name of the computer system that stores the information you seek, the directory path, and the pathname of the file comprising the pertinent page (such as /home.html). For example, "HTTP" is the protocol, or method of exchanging multimedia data, used by World Wide Web servers. (The initials stand for "HyperText Transport Protocol.") Some pathnames contain the character (˜) which designates a particular home directory on a server.

In some instances the same resource can be reached through more than one URL. URLs must be entered exactly as given and are case sensitive—upper and lower case letters must be used correctly. Though some URLs are very long, they must be entered as one continuous line with no spaces. For example, if your parent has any kind of disability, check out

http://www.eskimo.com/˜jlubin/usenet.html

Other URLs begin with
ftp://ftp
gopher://gopher
news:news.

COMMUNICATION

The communication side of the Internet is made up of various components. Here are some of them:

· *E-mail or Electronic Mail*—like the post office but faster, since it goes through your telephone and you don't have to wait for delivery. To use e-mail, you need an Internet address. It takes almost no time to learn how to compose, send, and receive mail.

- *Discussion Groups / Mailing List / Listservs*—These are specialized subscription lists for e-mail. They are restricted to members, who receive messages delivered to their e-mail address and send responses to fellow subscribers. Some lists have a moderator who reads incoming messages and decides whether they should be forwarded to the group. Most lists maintain archives of previous messages and other information of interest. There are many health-related mailing lists, or "listservs." Among them are listservs for Alzheimer's, cancer, diabetes, and Parkinson's (see p. 130 for more information).

- *Bulletin Board Systems (BBSs)*—These are another major thoroughfare for getting and sharing information. They are reached using standard communication software programs in your computer (such as ZTterm for Macintosh), plus a modem connected to a telephone. When you "dial up" a BBS, you connect your computer with a remote host. After the first connection, you can save the telephone number in your personal Internet phone directory located in the dial menu of your communication software.

Though few bulletin boards offer online conferencing, most offer "message boards" and access to database or program libraries. They provide excellent opportunities for online mutual help or access to particular interests. Users generally compose messages on their computer before they telephone the BBS. Then they dial up the BBS and send their message. Others call the BBS, read the messages, and send replies. Most BBSs are run from private homes. The person who runs a BBS is known as a "Sysop," or a systems operator. For example, "Osprey Nest" (modem phone connection: 301-989-9036) is the birdwatcher's bulletin board for Metropolitan Washington, D.C. "Senior Information on Line" (modem phone connection: 1-415-697-0520) offers information on healthcare and housing, leisure and recreation, financial and money matters.

· *Usenet Newsgroups*—"USENET" stands for "users network." This a network of 15,000 newsgroups each devoted to common interests, culled from both e-mail discussion groups and Listservs. Since it is not necessary to subscribe to read messages, and most newsgroups are unmoderated, audiences may be wider and messages more wide-ranging. Links to newsgroups require a World Wide Web software program that supports news-reading functions. You link through your Internet service provider. Like HTTP, news is the protocol for Usenet newsgroups.

Each newsgroup is divided into interest areas and arranged hierarchically within broad topic categories, using multipart names separated with periods. In USENET, the broad topics are:

comp (computer related topics)
rec (recreational and entertainment topics)
alt (alternative topics)
soc (social issues and political topics)
news (topics devoted to concerns of USENET); and
talk (forums for debate)

A sample newsgroup address is *alt.support.cancer.prostate.* As with message boards on commercial services or BBS, you can just read, or read and reply to, messages in each newsgroup.

· *Talk/Internet Relay Chats* are like the telephone, only you type in what you want to say. Unlike bulletin boards, these conversations take place in real-time. The commercial on-line services all have icons to enter public forums or chat groups. After signing into the service, you click the appropriate spot.

RESOURCES

The resource portion of the Internet is equally diverse. Resources can be programs, sound, pictures, documents, full-motion videos, and databases. The tools needed to access these resources—and to read, copy, and transfer their information—have their own acronyms: FTP, Telnet, Gopher, and WWW. They also have their own vocabulary such as "hosts," "login," and "pages."

INTERNET RESOURCE TOOLS

· File Transfer Protocol (FTP) allows you to retrieve programs or long documents (known as files) from computers around the network. Once you go to the FTP address (which begins with ftp://ftp) you will be asked to sign in. Most FTP sites are anonymous, meaning when you arrive at the site and are asked for a user name, you type "anonymous" and press OK. When asked for a password, type in your full Internet address. Then you will be logged in. To transfer or download files using FTP, you will learn about file types and how to convert the received information so your computer can read it. For example, some files are just text, while others are graphic; still others are special to IBM or MAC users.

· *Telnet* offers the ability to log onto a remote computer and navigate as if you were at the terminal of that computer. (Sometimes remote *hosts* require an account, asking you for an I.D. and a password. Others permit you to *log in* [sign on] as a guest or visitor without a password.)

· *Gopher*—This browsing tool helps you find, save (download), or print information found on the Internet. Gopher servers have main screens and menus (like the table of contents of a book) that help pull together scattered Internet text resources in a single, uniform format. They allow text-based information (for example, books, reports, articles, bibliographies) stored on one computer to be accessed by any other computer. The system, developed at the University of Minnesota (where the Golden Gophers are the football team), allows you to "go-pher" information from one computer site to another. For example, by typing in the Gopher URL of the catalog division of the Library of Congress, you are actually requesting connection to the main computer of the Library of Congress which houses that particular information.

Most Gopher sites are maintained by universities or other large organizations such as government agencies. Gophers were once the cutting edge of the Internet. But their limitation to words means they have taken a backseat to the more graphical World Wide Web.

An example of a Gopher address is the University of

Southern California Andrus Gerontology Center:
gopher://cwis.usc.edu/11/University__Information/
Academic__Departments/Gerontology

· *WorldWideWeb (WWW)*. The World Wide Web is a more advanced system of global information retrieval which overlays and supplements the connecting computer networks of the Internet. Gophers are used to find data through linear menus. Similarly, the key to the Web is a multidimensional menu—a powerful hypertext browsing system which allows the user both to *access* other Websites *beyond* the particular URL *and* investigate multimedia links to any selected word or phrase *within* a particular Website. If you visualize a site as a stack of pages, the "home page" is the top page. It holds the table of contents and is the place from which further links begin.

Unlike a Gopher, the table of contents on a Web home page can consist of graphics, sounds, and pictures as well as words. The content of individual Websites ranges from the text of a single document to those providing proprietary information and hundreds of links to other Websites. By 1996, the World Wide Web had *more than* forty million Web pages—up from 10,000 pages eighteen months before!

How do you use the Web? Through navigation software like Netscape's *Navigator* or Microsoft's *Internet Explorer,* which let your computer receive and examine any information contained in Web pages. Using point-and-click mouse commands and highlighted words, it is easy to scan the interlinked pages and retrieve related files containing text, images, or sound.

STEP 23—LOCATE RESOURCES WITH SEARCH TOOLS

The Internet and Web have each been described as a great library—with all the books spilled on the floor. *Archie, Veronica, Jughead,* and *WAIS* are Internet search and retrieval tools for putting those books in order—that is, for finding textual information on the Internet. Some search for strings of words; others use keywords.

- *Archie* is a database with over 2.5 million file names plus directories and sites where files are located. Archie helps you find specific files on FTP servers by name. You can telnet to Archie (using the username Archie) or send an e-mail to archie@archie.internic.net.

- *Veronica* uses keyword queries to locate titles listed by Gopher server.

- *WAIS* (Wide Area Information Server[s]) are huge databases that search by text of Gopher servers.

World Wide Web search engines help you explore the universe. They are interactive automated browsing tools, with names like *Lynx, Alta Vista, InfoSeek, Lycos,* and *Yahoo!* Some search for titles of documents. Others search the documents themselves. Still others use hierarchical indexes or directories. At the moment, most search engines are keyword-based; *Excite* has concept-based capabilities. This is particularly important when you realize how related terminology can vary. For example, if you search under "parentcare" you may find no entries, while the keyword "eldercare" may identify hundreds of options. It takes practice to learn how to search efficiently. But online instructions are available from each searching service.

- *Yahoo!* (Yet Another Hierarchical Officious Oracle) searches by category, topic, and word. The Yahoo! directory of Internet sites lists over 200,000 different resources indexed by 20,000 subject categories and subtopics.

- *Alta Vista* is one of the largest Web keyword indexes, covering eight billion words filling sixteen million pages. It offers simple or detailed searches for Web pages and 13,000 newsgroups.

- *Deja News* is a tool for searching Usenet. You can narrow your search by newsgroup, date, or author.

- *Excite* contains over a million Web documents and the most recent two weeks of Usenet news and classified ads. This service also provides NetReviews—sites evaluated for content quality—and news updates.

- *InfoSeek* is a free Web search service that scans web pages, newsgroups, usenet FAQs, and reviewed pages.

- *Lycos* sponsored by Carnegie-Mellon University is a text-search tool. is found in Netscape's search directory. It searches the Web by topic or keyword in titles, headings, links, or keywords of Web pages.

Step 24—Drive the Information Highway (With a Little Help from Your Friends)

Bulletin boards, ListServs, and Gopher addresses have been around for a decade. But the explosive introduction of the World Wide Web, cheaper, more powerful computers, faster modems, sophisticated search engines like Excite and Alta

Vista, user-friendly navigation software, and commercial on-line services—as well as new high-speed Integrated Services Digital Network (ISDN) telephone lines becoming available to residential users—have made the Internet much more accessible to millions of individuals with personal computers. For example, AT&T began offering direct "dial-up" nationwide Internet access to its eighty million residential and ten million business customers in March 1996. Half a million computer users signed up in the first month.

For caregivers or information seekers, Internet access may be as close as a neighbor, doctor, self-help organization, social worker, hospital, library, senior center, workplace, school, copy center, or shopping mall computer kiosk. Easy access to both equipment and a guide is not a dream. It's happening now, whether for free or a fee. Even "cybercafes" are cropping up around the country, with names like "Virtual Cafe," "@cafe" and "OnLine Cafe." In these shops customers can rent online computer time (at a going rate of $10 per hour) and surf the Net while they sip their tea.

If you are in a hurry, the easiest, cheapest, and fastest way to access the information highway is to tap the expertise and equipment of a friend, colleague, or information specialist familiar with your specific concern or the bells and whistles of the Internet. Not everyone has to learn to drive, especially if you can get there with someone else at the wheel. If that is your choice, then turn to p. 121 for information on Internet addresses and telephone numbers of a few key eldercare sites.

While all this sounds complicated, the process of using the internet and the Web to gather information is remarkably simple (see sample web page, p. 138).

Assuming you have found your way into the World Wide Web and a navigation software menu, choose the search icon.

Then select one of the search tools from the pop-up or pull-down menu (see Step 23, p. 109).

Next, type in a descriptive word or word string (which narrows the search to locate specific information). In seconds the search engine you have chosen sifts through its databases and creates on your screen an annotated list of related documents (in order of relevance) by title, Internet address (i. e., URL), and content.

If you have time, scroll through the entries until you find one you want. Or "save" or "print" the entire list for later reference.

Click on a highlighted word indicated by a bright color (hypertext) on this list, or type in the URL address, or click on a highlighted image representing the documents title. Any of these actions will zoom (hyperlink) you to the Web page of your choice—whether those sites are located across town or around the world.

Once at the new home page, you may scroll through a general table of contents, calling up material featured in hypertext by additional points and clicks—all without having to exit the document you started from.

When you are finished, click forward again to more in-depth information, or return to where you began. Graphical prompts on the computer screen show you how to go back through the entries you have chosen, save those you want for future reference, or print the information.

STEP 25—SELECT AN ACCESS RAMP TO THE INTERNET

PICKING A SERVICE

If you want to gather information through your computer at home, you will need some help getting hooked up to the Internet.

The process of making the computer, software, modem, and phone work together—the first time and every time—is still not perfect. You will need some technical support. There are many ways to get this help. You can stop in a bookstore or library and review an Internet guide, such as John R. Levine and Carol Baroudi's *The Internet for Dummies: The Beginner's Computer Guide.* You can hire a consultant to come to your home. You can sign up for local courses advertised in the newspaper. You could also visit more computer-savvy friends or sit down with your college-age children for a demonstration.

First you will need help finding (and connecting your computer modem to) an online "ramp." Here you have several choices. You can gain indirect access through a managed commercial network like America Online, CompuServe, or Prodigy. You can sign up for direct access with a community-based Freenet, major cable and telephone companies, or an Internet-only provider.

- *Commercial services*—America Online (phone: 1-800-827-9948), CompuServe (phone: 1-800-848-8199), and Prodigy (phone: 1-800-776-3449) are the "big three" of proprietary commercial computer networks. These national online services are like stand-alone electronic communities which provide gateway access to the Internet. They offer users the ability to read, post, and exchange messages in various specialty forums; search database libraries; and conference or "chat" with others in one-on-one or online meetings. These services provide their own software. They charge monthly fees for a minimum of five to ten hours, then bill for additional hours and services. All now provide varying access to the Internet and (as membership expands) growing support on parent care issues.

· *Freenets*—These are community-based networks in specific geographic areas. They provide free access to local information resources as well as selected topics of wider interest. Many larger Freenets provide e-mail, connections to Gophers, and access to other freenets. For example, there are freenets in Cleveland, Denver, East Central Illinois, Ottawa, Canada, and various public libraries. The Cleveland Freenet, working with local hospitals, sponsors online health clinics, health fairs, and health education seminars (modem phone connection: 216-368-3888).

· *Internet Service Providers*—If you like e-mail, enjoy surfing the World Wide Web or newsgroups, and find yourself spending over forty-five minutes online each day, it makes sense to investigate a hookup with a local or national access provider. In 1995, 3,200 such services were available, up from 1,800 the year before. These businesses operate special systems connected to the Internet and sell dial-up services ("hookups") for unlimited use for a flat monthly fee. You can choose between organized access or independent access, high use or low. AT&T, for example, offers customers unlimited monthly usage at $19.95. UUnet Technologies and PSINet offer comparable services.

Information about various service providers by state or area code, including their fees, services, phone, and fax numbers, can be found under the URL address: http://the list.com/.

There are two routes to direct Internet hookup: purchasing a software package, such as "Internet in a Box," or picking a service provider and using its Internet software. Either way, you will greatly benefit from technical assistance to help load your computer with appropriate graphic software and browsing programs.

QUESTIONS TO ASK

Maryland Internet consultant John Makulowich suggests that potential customers shopping for a direct access provider dial each provider's phone number at peak times (usually between 7 P.M. and 11 P.M.) to check for busy signals. If you cannot get through, choose another vendor. He also suggests asking any Internet provider:*

1. Do you have modem lines within a local call from my home?
2. What is the speed of your connection to the rest of the Internet?
3. What customer support and training do you offer?
4. How long have you been in business, and how many users do you currently support?
5. How often were your computers down last month?

*Source: *The Washington Post, Fast Forward Monthly Guide,* February 1996.

STEP 26—FIND TECHNICAL SUPPORT

Amazingly enough, all the technical help you will need is readily available. Much of it is free. For example, if you are already on line, consult your Internet provider's manual or collection of Frequently Asked Questions (known as "FAQs") posted on the network.

If you are nowhere near that stage, check the newspaper or telephone book for services such as those provided by Estelle Jacobs and Glorya Scherr, two enterprising seniors in Bethesda, Maryland. They run a company called "Training for the Terrified" aimed at the senior market. Their company teaches small classes or sends instructors to people at their homes. When Jacobs bought her first computer at age sixty-nine, she found she had to change her approach to her equipment:

> It wasn't that easy. . . . I thought it was sort of like a TV. You turn it on and it tells you what to do! . . . [I]t's more like buying a piano. Who would buy a piano without getting a piano teacher?*

There are other ways to learn about computers and online services. For example, Senior Net, a San Francisco-based national non-profit organization, is designed to introduce those over fifty-five to the joys of being online. With more than sixty centers across the country and 17,000 members, this group has an estimated 4,000 members online every day. There is a $35 annual fee. (Call 1-800-747-6848 and see p. 137 for more information.)

*"Seniors, Surfing the Net," *Washington Post,* October 3, 1995.

ELDERCARE AND THE INTERNET: POSSIBILITIES AND PITFALLS

STEP 27—ACCESS THE INTERNET FOR ELDERCARE INFORMATION

Telecommunications technology offers caregivers a great opportunity to overcome one of the most frustrating obstacles of effective eldercare—knowing that information and support services are available, but not knowing how to find them.

Cyberspace offers access to knowledge and resources as well as two-way communication. It enables eldercare consumers to learn about and manage care in advance of or even during a crisis. If you are facing imminent medical decisions, you can use the Gopher and World Wide Web systems to search medical libraries, review clinical trials, and download information on treatment and medication (see HyperDoc p. 129). You can also investigate thousands of newsgroups, review public access catalogs, and browse FTP, Gopher and World Wide Web sites for pertinent information from local, national, academic, government, commercial, and non-profit sources. Best of all, you can retrieve these materials to review at your leisure.

ELDERCARE COMMUNICATION THROUGH THE NET

Bulletin boards, Listservs, and e-mail offer consumers vast opportunities to combat isolation, reach out to others in similar circumstances, and tap common knowledge. Because participants are viewed solely through their messages or in real-time chat, the information highway is an equalizer, without social status or stigma. Users have anonymity; this often helps those uncomfortable sharing personal feelings. Because time and space are no longer constraints, online help is easily available to those in remote locations or to those who are bedridden.

Ed Madara, Director of the American Self-Help Clearinghouse has noted that online message exchanges resemble a self-help discussion group in slow motion. But unlike "real time mutual help, responses are usually carefully and thoughtfully prepared offline before being posted in response."

FINDING ELDERCARE RESOURCES THROUGH THE NET

Doctors, care managers, and eldercare information specialists pride themselves on "low-tech, high-touch" services. But they have traditionally reached patients or clients by telephone or in person. They are often inaccessible to caregivers who live far away or work regular jobs and can call only on evenings or weekends.

The information highway bypasses this barrier. It can deliver the whole world of products, services and care information direct to any networked home or workplace computer, day or night. As a result, caregivers, patients, doctors, researchers, and advocacy groups are using the Internet to address health and disease concerns. For example, publications of the Centers for Disease Control, the National Institute of Medicine, university research centers and advocacy groups all now have Internet sites.

CONSUMER BEWARE

What are the pitfalls? Two large ones: checking content and ensuring privacy. It is important to:

- Know the source of information in order to evaluate its quality and relevance.

- See who is responsible for data in the database.

- Note how frequently materials are updated.

- Verify that the message is posted by an "honest broker." The anonymity that encourages Internet speech also reduces responsibility for the content of that speech.

- Think about confidentiality before transmitting any personal information.

- Take care before buying any product online.

STEP 28—SEARCH THE INTERNET WITH THE ELDERCARE KEYWORD INDEX (P. 265)

Language barriers also impede access to eldercare information on the information highway, though they are easier to overcome. The problems remain lack of standard terms and too much information, rather than too little. For example, searchers may be handicapped by the absence of a common term to describe the general topic of helping to care for parents. Start with the keywords "Eldercare," "Aging," or "Seniors" to locate General Sites or SuperSites on related eldercare and aging issues. Or select the web search engine Yahoo! and type in the keyword "Health" for a list of specific conditions. Scroll to the latest information about specific diseases (see Health Care, p. 129). Then you can link to additional information on research, treatment, diet, and support (see Alzheimer's, p. 131). Material on long-term care insurance, for instance may be found under "insurance," "money and finance," or "healthcare."

To find specific information, use the keywords identified in the Keyword Index of this book (p. 265) along with the powerful Internet search and browsing tools. You will find navigating the Net much easier than relying on the library card catalog, the telephone book, or friends. Some examples are "Elder Law" (see p. 128), "Managed Care" (see p. 133), "Assisted Living" (see p. 133), "Home Health Care" (see p. 132), and specific health conditions. These are your "shazams" to get information online. You will be amazed at what you learn.

STEP 29—CREATE A "HOT LIST" OF WEB ADDRESSES

It may take a few years before all service providers, especially those from the non-profit world, make their information available in an ordinary fashion on the Internet and the World Wide Web. But each provider does not need an individual page for you to learn about their services. For example, you can find useful eldercare Websites maintained by a local government agency, a non-profit group, a city newspaper, or a taskforce of working caregivers. (See Caregivers on p. 125 of the following guide.) When you mark the site for saving, and check back at a later time for new resources, be sure to press the "reload" button, so you get updated information on your computer.

See Appendix 3 for a summary of Eldercare Internet Addresses.

A SAMPLER OF ELDERCARE INTERNET ADDRESSES

RESOURCES

INTERNET AND E-MAIL RESOURCES ON AGING

- **URL: http://www.aoa.dhhs.gov/aoa/pages/jpostlst.html**
Compiled by Joyce Post, librarian, Philadelphia Geriatric Center, Philadelphia, Pennsylvania (updated May, 1996).
DESCRIPTION: Annotated list of 639 items. Twenty-two cross-referenced sections include:

- Aging, aging research
- Alzheimer's disease, dementia, and related disorders
- Associations, conferences
- Biosciences, neurobiology
- Caregiving
- Consumer topics
- Demographic centers, datasets, and statistical information

- Education
- Finances and economics
- Government agencies and organizations (national)
- Health
- Information services and centers, libraries, data-bases
- Intergenerational relation-ships
- Legal

- Living arrangements, nursing homes, retirement communities
- Long-term care industry, long-term care administration
- Meeting places for seniors
- Nursing
- Psychology, psychiatry
- Retirement
- Special populations
- State and local services, agencies, and resources

ADMINISTRATION ON AGING HOME PAGE

- **URL: http://www.aoa.dhhs.gov**

Compiled by Saadia Greenberg, Staff, U.S. Administration on Aging (AoA), Washington, D.C.

DESCRIPTION: Information about the Administration on Aging and its programs, resources for practitioners, statistical information on the aging population, and information for consumers, including how to obtain services and electronic booklets on aging-related issues.

DIRECTORY OF WEB AND GOPHER AGING SITES

- **URL: http://www.aoa.dhhs.gov/aoa/webres/craig.htm**

Compiled by Bruce Craig, Staff, U.S. Administration on Aging, Washington, D.C.

DESCRIPTION: Contains an Internet index of Area Agencies on Aging, and a directory of other Internet Aging Sites.

GENERAL SITES FOR CAREGIVERS AND SENIORS (Alphabetical)

BLACKSBURG ELECTRONIC VILLAGE SENIOR INFORMATION (BEV)

● **URL: http://www.bev.net/community/seniors/**
*Developed by senior citizen subscribers of the BEV "Seniors
Electronic Mailing List."*
BEV-SENIORS@LISTSERV.VT.EDU
DESCRIPTION: An experiment to enhance computer com-
munications among seniors connecting an entire Virginia
town to the Internet. Contents include letters to the editor; senior members and profiles; merchant discounts;
links to other senior sites; government resources; local
programs; and financial information.

CAREGIVERS

● **URL: http://www.sfgate.com/examiner/caregivers series**
San Francisco Examiner *senior editor Beth Witrogen McLeod's
"Caregivers" series April 2–9, 1995.*
DESCRIPTION: Stories on caregivers, finding housing; finan-
cial worries; hospice care; and adult day care.

ELDERCARE WEB

● **URL: http://www.ice.net/~kstevens/ELDERWEB.HTM**
Created by Karen Stevenson Brown, CPA, Normal, Illinois
DESCRIPTION: Eldercare information for both providers
and consumers. Hypertext to hundreds of documents and
dozens of sites including the National Health Information
Center database, MedWeb (Emory University Health Sci-

ences Center Library). Sections include health care; living arrangements; death and dying; social; mental and spiritual; financial; law and legislation; statistics and demographics; state-specific information; and a provider locator.

INSTITUTE OF GERONTOLOGY
- **URL: http://www.iog.wayne.edu**

Service of the Institute of Gerontology, Wayne State University, Detroit, Michigan

DESCRIPTION: Online resource for researchers, educators, practitioners, and those interested in the concerns of senior citizens.

CONTENTS: *GeroWeb,* featuring the "Virtual Library on Aging;" links to gerontology and geriatric sites; *Division 20,* a website of the American Psychological Association's branch devoted to adult development and aging; *Michigan Aging Services,* with information about services for Michigan's seniors; a calendar of events; and information on continuing education.

SENIOR.COM
- **URL: http://www.senior.com**

Commercial site, created by Tom Poole, businessman and caregiver, Seattle, Washington

DESCRIPTION: Home page arranged as a "town square" with point-and-click buildings for Prime Lifestyles; Travel, City Hall; Health and Professional Services; and Gus's NewsStand.

CONTENT: Public information and commercial products and services. Focus is on the interests of active as well as more frail seniors. Features include information; message centers; and chat groups.

SELECTED STATE AND COMMUNITY RESOURCES ON THE INTERNET

CAREGIVERS RESOURCE GUIDE

● **URL: http://www.sfgate.com/examiner/caregivers/resources/national.html**
SOURCE: *San Francisco* Examiner, *San Francisco, California*
CONTENTS: How to Find Help: San Francisco; Alameda County; Contra Costa County; Marin County; Santa Clara County; San Mateo County; Solano and Napa Counties; National Organizations; bibliography; and online resources

CHICAGO DEPARTMENT ON AGING

● **URL: http://www.ci.chi.il.us/WorksMart/Aging/**
SOURCE: *Local Government Agency*
DESCRIPTION: Rated first in quality of Website content of Area Agencies on Aging by the Administration on Aging "Directory of Web and Gopher Sites." Links to local programs and services such as benefits eligibility; carrier alert; housing; disability; chore/housekeeping; employment; foster grandparents; nutrition; life enrichment; volunteers; medical transport; protective services; respite care; and senior companions.

CLEVELAND FREENET—A PUBLIC ACCESS NETWORK

MODEM CONNECTION: Telnet to: freenet-in-b.cwru.edu
Log in as either "guest" or "visitor;" at the prompt for type of access type: 2; at the prompt type: GO ALZ, then "5." The best time to call is from 11 P.M. to 8 A.M. EST.

1. Alzheimer's Disease Support Center (ADSC)

SPONSORS: *Case Western Reserve University and the Cleveland Area chapter of the Alzheimer's Association, Cleveland, Ohio.*

DESCRIPTION: A Telnet Internet resource. Offers training and assistance to caregivers in computer setup and system use as well as a number of free computers for caregivers.

CONTENT: Modules on communication, professional advice, and information. Includes publications and audiovisuals, information on caregiver support group meetings, and a calendar of events. Community Resource Directory includes information on assisted living; bereavement; case management; day care centers; emergency response systems; home care; geriatric assessment; legal services; nursing homes with special care units; physicians; senior centers; and short-stay respite programs.

DIRECTORY OF ST. LOUIS RESOURCES FOR SENIORS

- **URL: http://www.riversidepavillion.com/dirorg.html**
SOURCE: *Riverside Pavillion Skilled Nursing Facility. Prepared by Rick Troupin.*

CONTENT: A community resources directory includes thirty cross-references to specific information including in-home services, housing, grief support groups, and long-term care management.

PRINCETON UNIVERSITY ELDERCARE CONTACT RESOURCE GUIDE

- **URL: http://www.princeton.edu/Main/elder.html**
COMPILER: *Maryann Arnold, Flex/Time/Childcare Task Force of the Committee on the Status of Women and Office of Human*

Resources for faculty and staff at Princeton University, Princeton, New Jersey.

DESCRIPTION: A guide to local eldercare services for five Pennsylvania and New Jersey counties around Princeton. Lists telephone numbers and addresses of national, state, and county eldercare health, self-help, and service organizations. Includes services such as adult day care; caregiver support; emergency aid; financial aid; food/meal programs; homemaker health services; hospices, housing rent assistance; housing repair; information and referral; insurance assistance and information; legal assistance; recreation; relative reassurance; respite care; transportation; and volunteer opportunities.

SPECIFIC TOPICS (Listed Alphabetically)

COPING SKILLS
- **URL: http://asa.ugl.lib.umich.edu/chdocs/support/emotion.html**
    1. Emotional Support Guide
Prepared by Johanne Juhnke and Chris Powell, School of Information and Library Studies, University of Michigan.
DESCRIPTION: "Internet Resources for Physical Loss, Chronic Illness and Bereavement." Chronic Illness resource by subject (such as AIDS, Arthritis, Diabetes, Multiple Sclerosis, Parkinson's disease, and Prostate Cancer). Resources indexed by title and Internet tool.

DISABILITY

- **URL: http://.pulver.com/netwatch/topten**

  1. NetWatch Top Ten—Net Access for Disabled

  AUTHOR: *Kevin Price, University of Missouri-Columbia ACT Center*
  Top ten sites include the one listed below.

- **URL: http://disability.com**

  2. Disability Resources on the Internet

  SOURCE: *Commercial. Evan Kemp Associates of Capital Heights, Maryland provides Disability Resources, Products and Services.*
  DESCRIPTION: A comprehensive site on general resources. Fourteen categories link to hundreds of sites with information on careers and jobs; government resources; Internet information; medicine/health; non-profits; recreation/entertainment/lifestyle information; universities/education; and Visual/Hearing.

ELDER LAW

- **URL: http://ukanaix.cc.ukans.edu/~webmom/ keln—main.html**

  1. Kansas Elder Law Network (KELN)

  Maintained by Kim Dayton, Law Professor, University of Kansas, (affiliated with University of Kansas Elder Law Clinic).
  DESCRIPTION: A public service site for state and national community. Table of Contents includes bulletins; index to annotated bibliographies of elder law practice; index to KELN legal databases; links to other Web sites in health resources; government agencies and laws; legal assistance and advocacy; and statistical information. Includes a guide to legal resources on the Web.

GOVERNMENT INFORMATION

- **URL: http://www.fedworld.gov**

    1. FedWorld Information Network
SOURCE: *Compiled by the National Technical Information Services (NTIS), to help access U.S. Government Information online. Washington, D.C.*
DESCRIPTION: A comprehensive central access point for locating and acquiring government information. Goal is to provide one-stop location for the public. Connects to other government Websites and dial-in bulletin boards.

- **URL: http://www.loc.gov**

    2. Library of Congress
Washington, D.C.
DESCRIPTION: General information and publications; government congress and law; research and collections services; copyright; access to Library of Congress online services including databases and catalog or connection to the library's Gopher; and events and exhibits. Topical collections of Internet resources are organized by Library of Congress subject specialists.

HEALTH CARE

- **URL: http://www.nlm.nih.gov/(NLM)**
- **URL: http://igm.nlm.nih.gov/(Grateful med)**

    1. HyperDocMed
National library of medicine online information services
SOURCE: *Prepared for the National Center for Biotechnology Information, Bethesda, Maryland.*
DESCRIPTION: Health research online via link to MED-LARS, the vast computer system of the National Library of

Medicine's (NLM) eighteen million references. MEDLARS (MEDical Literature Analysis and Retrieval System) is a system of databases and databanks related to biomedical research and patient care. NLM's GRATEFUL MED software offers user-friendly access to most of them. Available databases include MEDLINE with references and abstracts to journal articles, DIRLINE, a directory of information resources online, and CANCERLIT, with references to cancer literature. A Bulletin Board System links the NLM and users of GRATEFUL MED to Clinical Alerts highlights from the National Institute of Health's (NIH) clinical trials and is easily available.

To search under the Grateful Med gateway, you need to obtain a user I.D. code/password and complete an order form for the $29.95 software. You can do this online or by calling the National Library of Medicine, 8600 Rockville Pike, Bethesda, Maryland 20894. (phone: 1-800-638-8480; e-mail: mms@nlm.nih.gov.) A detailed users guide gives specific information on the user costs and capabilities of the system. It shows you how to log on, do a search, and cross-reference searches. You can print what you have found and download the information. You can also order hardcopy of documents.

- **URL: http://www.yahoo.com/Health**
  2. Search Engine: *Yahoo—Health:*
  Category "Health" listings include: Alternative Medicine; Death and Dying; Diseases and Conditions; Fitness; Geriatrics and Aging; Health Care; Health Insurance; Nutrition; Sexuality; and Travel.
  Searching here, you will find links to:

ALZHEIMER'S DISEASE AND DEMENTIA

To subscribe send a message to:

MAJORDOMO@WUBIOS.WUSTL.EDU

Leave the subject line blank; send a one line message:subscribe ALZHEIMER (no name). To send a message or reply to the list after you are a subscriber use:

ALZHEIMERS@WUBIOS.WUSTL.EDU

Archives messages posted:

- **URL: http://www.biostat.wustl.edu/alzheimer/**
- **URL: gopher://gopher.ardc.wustl.edu/**

    1. Alzheimer's List/Serve

SPONSOR: *Washington University Alzheimer's Disease Research Center.*

DESCRIPTION: For professionals, caregivers, students, or anyone with an interest in Alzheimer's disease. Active caregiver discussion group.

- **URL:**

  http://www.biostat.wush.edu/ALZHEIMER/submit.html

    2. Alzheimer Page—Web Links on Aging and
       Dementia

SOURCE: *Alzheimer's Disease Research Center of Washington University at St. Louis, Missouri.*

DESCRIPTION: Hyperlinks caregiver resources; clinical care guides; research discussions; commercial products and services; job listings; personal home pages; nursing homes/assisted living. Following the trail of this site, you can link to Web pages in foreign countries, all for the price of a local call.

● **URL: http://www.alz.org**

    3. Alzheimer's Association (U.S.)

SOURCE: *Non-profit Alzheimer's Association has 35,000 volunteers, 221 local chapters and 2,000 support groups nationwide. Based in Chicago, Illinois.*

DESCRIPTION: In addition to recent news on the disease, this site has general information, a location map for local chapters, caregiver resources, medical information, and content on public policy. There are links to other Alzheimer's Websites plus a search engine for Alzheimer's-related documents.

HOME CARE

● **URL: http://www.traverse.com/health/mhhc/home.html**

    1. In Home Help—Michigan Home Health Care

SOURCE: *Information page of two rural Northern Michigan home health agencies—Michigan Home Health Care and In Home Help.*

DESCRIPTION: Hyperlinks to consumer information about home healthcare services; hospice; how to choose a home health agency; payment questions; and health and disease links.

● **URL: http://www.nahc.org/**

    2. National Association for Home Care (NAHC)

SOURCE: *Web page of the trade association of 7,000 Home Care Agencies.*

DESCRIPTION: Information on membership services, conferences, news and information, legislative and regulatory issues, FAQs and consumer information about home care and hospice. Hypertext topics include "How to Choose a Home Care Agency," "A Listing of Home Care and Hos-

pice State Associations," "Background on Home Care,"
"Statistics on Home Care," and "The Hospice Patient's Bill
of Rights."

HOUSING
- **URL: http:www.seniorsites.com**
    1. Senior Sites
SOURCE: *Posted by the California Association of Homes and
Services for the Aging, Sacramento, California.*
DESCRIPTION: Contains a reference guide of non-profit
providers of senior housing; healthcare and services; a full-
text searchable listing of non-profit providers; and a list of
national and state organizations.

- **URL: gopher://gopher.gsa.gov:70/00/staff/pa/cic/
health/nursehme.txt**
    2. "Guide to Choosing a Nursing Home"
    Online publication of the Health Care Financing Adminis-
    tration (HCFA)
DESCRIPTION: Excellent "first step" booklet guides families
on places to go, people to speak with and some questions to
ask. Offers information on payment considerations, long-
term care insurance, and a checklist of features to consider.

INSURANCE
- **URL: http://www.ncqa.org**
    1. National Committee for Quality Assurance (Managed
    Care)
SOURCE: *An independent not-for-profit organization which
assesses and reports on the quality of managed care plans,
including HMOs. Seeks to help consumers distinguish among*

plans to make better decisions. Organization focused on
accrediting and performance measurement criteria.
CONTENTS: Links to information on accreditation; performance report cards; conferences; and publications.

LONG-TERM CARE
- **URL: http://www.housecall.com**
  1. America's HouseCall Network (AHCN) Older Adult
     Resources Forum (Under Development)

SOURCE: *Under the umbrella of the Orbis Broadcast Group,*
America's HouseCall Network is a healthcare information and
education system. The Older Adult Resources Forum is made up of
an alliance of aging organizations including the American Society
on Aging, the SPRY foundation and the National Meals on Wheels
Foundation.

DESCRIPTION: Comprehensive information on medical and
nonmedical long-term care services for older adults and
their families and the professionals serving them. Content
on health; caregiving; housing; nutrition; financial issues;
and home and community-based services.

MEDICARE
- **URL: http:hcfa.gov/medicare/medicare.html**
  1. Medicare

SOURCE: *The Health Care Financing Administration (HCFA) is*
part of the U.S. Department of Health and Human Services and
is responsible for administration of both Medicare and Medicaid
programs.

CONTENT: Information about HCFA; Medicare; Medicaid;
regulations; statistics; research; publications; forms; and
links to other government servers.

MEDICATION

- **URL: http://pharminfo.com/pin–hp.html**
    1. PharmInfo Net

SOURCE: *Service provided by VirSci Corporation, a company not associated with any pharmaceutical company.*

DESCRIPTION: The Pharmaceutical Information Network contains a wide range of documents and databases such as Publications; Drug InfoBase; Medical InfoBase; PharMall; Pharmacy Corner; and PharmLinks. The contents of PharmLinks include resources on drug information; research and development; general pharmaceutical resources; government resources; medical resource links; pharmacy associations; pharmacy schools and educational resources; and information on pharmaceutical companies.

SOCIAL SECURITY

- **URL: http://www.ssa.gov/programs/programs–intro.html**
    1. Social Security Online

SOURCE: *Social Security Administration (SSA).*

DESCRIPTION: Index includes information about the Social Security Administration, its history, retirement, survivors, disability, and SSI programs; customer service standards; information on processing disability applications; FAQs; finances; forms; GILS (Government Information Locator Services); legislation; policy; public information resources; rulings; research and statistical data.

SAMPLE AGING RELATED DISCUSSION GROUPS/LISTSERVS

- **URL: http://tile.net/tile/cgi-bin/gerinet.html**
    1. GERINET

A General listserv

To subscribe send a message to:
LISTSERV@UBVM.CC.Buffalo.EDU; leave the subject
line blank; send a one line message:subscribe GERINET
(firstname lastname). To send a message or reply to the list
after you are a subscriber use:
GERINET@ubvm.cc.buffalo.edu

Bulletin Board Systems
   1. AGENET

SOURCE: *National Association of State Units on Aging,
Washington, D.C.*

CONTENTS: Four databases, three of which are biblio-
graphic. Call the BBS at 1-800-989-2243 (8 bits and 1 stop
bit). Give your name and select a password. Menus will
guide you through online session. See Also: Bruce
Maxwell, *How to Access the Government's Bulletin Boards,*
(Congressional Quarterly Books), describing the 200
federal BBSs that offer free access to information.

COMMERCIAL ONLINE SERVICES

America Online (AOL) (phone: 1-800-827-9948)
- **URL: http://www.seniornet.com.**
   1. **AARP On-line.** News, information, and interactive
      communications with articles from the AARP Bulletin,
      AARP information brochures, consumer "chat" groups,
      and software exchange. Information on Medicaid;
      Medicare; caregiving; estate planning; and senior hous-
      ing. AARP members receive reduced rates to subscribe
      to AOL. AOL subscribers do not have to be AARP

members to enter this site. Type keyword "AARP" after logging on (also available on CompuServe and Prodigy).

2. **Caregiving and Aging: Issues and Concerns.** Topics range from arthritis and bath lifts to getting your affairs in order, hypothermia, patient lifts, and stroke. Type keyword "Health."

3. **SeniorNet On-line.** SeniorNet is a non-profit group with 17,000 members and 75 computer centers throughout the United States to teach computer skills to seniors. Joint partnership with the Gray Panthers and the Older Women's League. After paying AOL monthly fees, SeniorNet members (who pay a membership fee) receive unlimited time on SeniorNet On-line; AOL nonmembers can also access SeniorNet On-line. Type Keyword "SeniorNet."

4. *Additional Keywords: "Senior," "DisAbilities," and "Consumers"*

COMPUSERVE (PHONE: 1-800-848-8199)

1. *Retirement Living Forum.*
Managed by Jeff Finn, Director, Setting Priorities for Retirement Years (SPRY) Foundation.
Forum contains a message/bulletin board, a topical library, and a Conference Center. Library keywords are organized by activity (caregiving) rather than condition (Alzheimer's). Subscribers can browse through documents, read them, and print for personal use. Conferences with subject-area experts. Subscribers may participate "live" in the session, or leave a question and check in later for a response. (See also House Call p. 134) Keyword: "Go RETIRE" after logging on to CompuServe.

- URL: http://www.ssa.gov/programs/programsintro.html

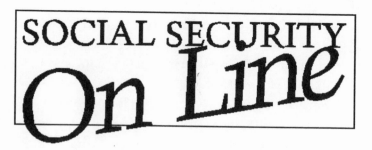

Welcome to **Social Security Online**, a service of the Social Security Administration, maintained by the Team Internet and part of our Agency's commitment to the goal of providing World Class Service.

Please use our feedback form to help us provide better service to you. We would like to have your comments and suggestions about **Social Security Online.** Because the Internet is not secure, we request that you **not** include any personal information, especially Social Security numbers, in your feedback. Questions about individual claims should be directed to 1-800-772-1213. Also, please be aware that Social Security records are confidential and we are prohibited from releasing information, including the whereabouts, on any living person.

For quick access to information, see our Frequently Asked Questions (FAQs) or see our How Do I? files.

QUICK INDEX

Agency Information I Benefit Information I Customer Service Standards I Disability Process Redesign I En Español I FAQs IFinances I Forms I GILS I Guide for Employers I How Do I? I International I Legislation I Local Office Information I Other Servers of Interest I Policy Forum I Public Information Resources I Rulings I Research and Statistics I Satellite Broadcasts I Search I Site Map I

WHAT'S NEW

The information on this server was last updated on May 1, 1996.

Request Your Earnings and Benefit Estimate Statement Here

PART THREE

MAKING

DECISIONS

HELPING YOUR PARENTS MAKE DECISIONS

Jumping to conclusions about what is best for your parents—paying little attention to their desires and inclinations—weakens their confidence and diminishes their capabilities. Your task in decision making is just the opposite: to strengthen their capabilities through effective support. While the degree of your involvement may vary over time, there are two types of decisions to consider. The first involves preventive measures against the unexpected. The second involves parents' safety and welfare. Steps 30 through 42 will help guide you through the process.

In today's complex world, it is necessary to take preventive measures against events such as medical catastrophe, impoverishment, or incapacity which you hope may never happen. Even if your parents' health is good now, it may not stay that way. Using common sense, you should expect that at some time in the future your parents may need much more care, or even total care, which they may not be able to afford.

Preparing a strategy for this possibility takes time and energy; it involves listening to professional advice and reading a lot of small print. Your willingness to dig through the technical sludgepiles of Medicare and Medicaid eligibility requirements, insurance policies, and legal forms offers some assurance that if catastrophe does strike, your parents will have some protection. These nitty-gritty concerns will be covered in more detail on pages 149–96.

Your parents' decisions about moving or not revolve around safety and care arrangements. Should your parents want to stay in their home as long as possible, you can help them remove household hazards, make their home more accessible, and get additional help while they remain in place— critical measures determining their comfort, independence, and quality of life. These decisions are largely, but not exclusively, framed by money, technology, and available human resources.

You may know what resources parents have to draw on. But do you know how much money is enough? Or how it can be used to greatest advantage? You know how much your parents can do and want to do. But do you know how today's technology can help maintain their independence? You know the many demands on your own life. But do you know how to meet the demands on your parents' lives—how, for instance, to bridge the gaps between what they need and what you can provide, with services provided by others? Aspects of safety and welfare are discussed on pages 197–218 and housing options on pages 218–29.

Before getting too specific about decision making, let's discuss for a moment what it may be like to work things out with your parents. In assembling documents and financial records you probably met at least some resistance. So don't be surprised if any conversation with your parents that suggests a change of lifestyle—no matter what the "objective advantage" or "added convenience" from *your* perspective—

seems to go back and forth with no conclusion. This carousel is often deceptive. Things may be progressing more smoothly than you think.

In some cases your *parents'* judgment of what is right for them and *your* judgment of what is right for them may differ. This does not mean one of you is wrong. Sometimes—indeed, quite often—the difference of opinion flows from different attitudes, perceptions, or philosophies.

For example, when you and your parents discuss the financial information you have helped them gather, you may draw opposite conclusions from the same facts. The amount of money they have will be indisputable, and you may be relieved to discover they are financially well off. But they may see the poorhouse around the corner. Your respective attitudes toward the future, and your respective judgments about the potential costs of their future care, will likely account for your differing views.

Approaches to spending money may also differ. Your parents may enjoy finding techniques to stretch dollars, but promptly spend what they save on items to add more fun or style to their lives.

Perhaps they are "what, me worry?" types who calculated thirty years ago how much they needed for a comfortable cushion, accumulated it through savings and investments and now cannot see that the world has changed, making their plan a formula for disaster. Or they may have devoted so many years to accumulating wealth that now they are unable to switch to the necessary spending mode. Perhaps they have become benefactors, spreading their wealth around, more concerned about their children and their children's children than their own future. Or they may procrastinate, never making final choices, always poised for decision but delay-ing that binding step.

You and your parents may even disagree about capa-bilities. For example, if you are worried about your parents' ability to manage at home, you may want them to hire a housekeeper to spend a few hours each day with them. From your perspective, this step can maintain their independence and provide some security. From theirs, it may be injecting "a stranger into the house."

Parents may acknowledge they need some help getting dressed, taking out the trash, preparing meals, cleaning, shopping, driving, taking medication, doing taxes, or filing health claims. Yet they may welcome *your* assistance but balk at any "outside meddling," especially if they have never del-egated these tasks. They may argue strangers will steal the silver or jewelry. They may resent intrusions on their privacy as unnecessary and expensive, and groan about paying good money for "just having someone around . . . to babysit."

On the other hand, your approach itself may be a real ob-stacle. After all, your parents are like you and your chil-dren—only more so. They resent being told what to do or when to do it. Older people tend to fear the future, espe-cially if it looks unpleasant. Often they deny how close the future is.

Through your efforts you may gather drawers of infor-mation, catalogs of gadgets, and books of backup systems—only to see these options rejected while your parents cling to the status quo and wait for the most recent crisis to sub-side.

As you go about helping (and sometimes acting) on your

parents' behalf, keep in mind that you, the adult children, may have *influence.* But you have limited *authority.* If your parents are managing alone (whether they think they can and you disagree, or they think they cannot and you still disagree), as long as they are capable of making their own decisions, you will have to step back and let them act. If they are in the driver's seat, they are the ones who must drive.

Do what you can, but prepare yourself and your parents to accept the fact that guilty as you may feel—and angry as they may act—you cannot prevent, anticipate, arrange for, or meet their every need.

You are dealing with your parents, not your children. You do not want—and they do not want you—to reverse roles and become their parent. If you view them as dependent and childlike, and place yourself in the parent role, you will only arouse conflicting emotions of anxiety, resentment, anger, and guilt. And you will end up with negative results. So you cannot give orders or expect instant obedience.

If giving orders is your style, expect stiff resistance and prepare for resentment and anger. If you demand that your parents do something and they say "No, we won't!" there's little you can do. In Herb Gardner's superb play *I'm Not Rappaport,* the concerned daughter of the decrepit elderly hero presents him with three "nonnegotiable" options: live with her in suburbia, move to a total care facility, or attend daily a senior center with hours of stupefying sessions on crafts and health care. He munches his dentures. "I see," he says. "It's either Siberia, Devil's Island . . . or kindergarten." And stays right where he is.

No one likes to lose control. And no one likes situations

which emphasize or exaggerate that loss. Out of love and trust, your parents may have turned to you for emotional support. They fear dependency, helplessness, and the reduced status they face with each disability. They are angry at their body's betrayal, about the state of their health, perhaps at needing you to be more attentive. They may fight getting old and needing help. They fear being a burden. And they are almost certain to resist or resent your taking over. Remind yourself that your task is to strengthen their capabilities with your support, not weaken them by your interference. Logic, common sense, even love are your weapons.

When conflicts arise, listen to what your parents are really saying. Acknowledge their point of view. Then listen to yourself. Then try again, explaining first the impact their actions (or lack of actions) are having on your own life. If you can only disagree with what parents are or are not doing (or if you do not like what is happening to them), back off. Exercise restraint. Limit yourself to what you expected from them when you moved away and began your own independent life.

There are other parental reactions to anticipate. For example, if your father is able to leave the house and wants social and intellectual stimulation, he may enjoy part-time work, volunteer activities, continuing education programs, or exercise classes at senior centers or health clubs. But he may also be reluctant to commit to any of these. He may need a boost to get going.

Your parents' attitude also makes a big difference. It is tough enough to cope as the body's machinery wears down. Impediments or illness do not make the job easier. But parents respond differently to similar limitations. Some welcome every ramp, wheelchair, elevator, handicapped parking place, gadget, and device, recognizing the benefit of enhanced autonomy. Others will not admit they can benefit from these conveniences and shun their perceived "stigma," insisting such devices are only for those "worse off." A third group may be aware of the benefits, but view with loathing all special license plates, wheelchairs, canes, and gadgets, rejecting such "proof" of physical deterioration.

If your parents fit the second and third description, you may suffer as you watch them struggle. But consider their view of the same battles to shop, get to the doctor, manage finances, climb steps. They may see these acts as defiantly life-affirming, not debilitating. They may view accommodation of adversity as a personal defeat rather than a triumph.

Finally, since your parents are at a different stage of life than you, your respective reaction times will be different. You may find it easy to switch gears and flexibly adapt to rapidly changing circumstances. They may find even the prospect of change terrifying. If your parents' response to your suggestions is consistently negative, reexamine your timetable. They know best where and how hard the shoe pinches. They simply may need more time to adjust.

In most cases, by talking through these differences you and your parents will be able to find common ground and reach a consensus on important decisions. But in some cases you will reach an impasse. They will want to go in one direction, you would like them to go in another. And some choices cannot be split down the middle. Expect this to happen from time to time. Just remind yourself that your parents are adults, ultimately responsible for their own lives. When their choice goes against your judgment, do not pick up your marbles and go home. Hang in there and work with your parents on the next decision. You and they are not two opposing teams; no one is keeping score, and this is not a game of win or lose. You are a family.

TAKING PREVENTIVE MEASURES

Our parents provided for our needs when we were growing up. Now we must make sure they are equally protected.

To be on the safe side, it is *absolutely necessary* to make provisions which shield your parents and yourself against catastrophe, impoverishment, and incapacity. This means two types of tasks: finding the right insurance, and putting the right kind of legal documents in place. Since the basic legal and insurance issues are fairly common, you will discover many "experts" on the merits and demerits of various options. These include legal or financial professionals; friends; neighbors or relatives; and strangers you will deal with by telephone at the Social Security Office, Area Office on Aging, social service organizations, or membership groups such as unions or the American Association of Retired Persons (AARP).

There are a lot of sources of good advice out there. Ask, listen, and follow up; you will save time, money, and aggravation.

As you will see, one set of tasks necessary to protect your parents involves being a good consumer when shopping for insurance. Another involves taking specific legal and financial measures to protect your parents' wishes in the event of incapacity. The backup materials for these decisions are both grim and dry. If you do not need to collect them now, just skim the contents below. You can come back later, when you need details. In a sense, what follows is a series of "buyer beware" warnings—designed to leave your parents more protected and more in control.

PREVENT CATASTROPHE WITH HEALTH INSURANCE

To be an informed consumer of health insurance takes time, energy and effort. The step-by-step process involves gathering information, learning the basics of Medicare, studying various plans, evaluating options, considering alternatives if parents have limited income and assets, comparison shopping, and decision making.

There are many choices, and comparing options is often difficult because of the specific health needs, age, and financial position of your parents. Steps 30, 31, and 32 will help you do the following:

- Learn about Medicare's basic coverage and gaps
- Study the ten standard Medigap plans and managed care plans.
- Compare only the policies that meet your needs.
- Consider alternatives if your parents have limited income.
- Contact your state health insurance counseling program for information.

STEP 30—LEARN MEDICARE'S COVERAGE AND LIMITS. FIND OUT WHO PAYS FOR HOSPITAL, NURSING HOME, OR HOME CARE, AND FOR HOW LONG

If your parents are over sixty-five (or under sixty-five and disabled) and eligible for Social Security, they are entitled to hospital and medical insurance coverage under Medicare. Medicare is the federal fee-for-service insurance program officially known as "Health Insurance for the Aged and Disabled." Title XVIII, the Social Security Act, was enacted in 1965 to provide healthcare for those least likely to have access to private health insurance because of age and preexisting conditions.

There is no question Medicare has been a blessing for the elderly. It currently pays almost 70 percent of their hospital costs and 60 percent of their doctor bills. But its cost is high and growing higher as the U.S. population ages and expensive medical technologies emerge. Medicare is supposed to be, and is, an umbrella against ruinous health costs. But this umbrella offers both more and less rainy-day protection than you may think.

In 1995 the Medicare program had thirty-six million enrollees, 90 percent of them over age sixty-five. That year Medicare spent $176 billion—18 percent of total health spending in the United States. Americans spend enormous sums of money at the end of life. For example, over 27 percent of Medicare expenses comes from care for the 5.9 percent of the Medicare population that dies each year. For those admitted to hospitals, Medicare spends six times as much on a person who dies as on one who lives.

There is a great misunderstanding about Medicare coverage. The U.S. Health Care Financing Administration (HCFA) administers the Act, and through local Social Security offices you can call the Medicare Hotline (1-800-638-6833) to order such valuable information HCFA pamphlets as *Your Medicare Handbook,* the *Guide to Health Insurance for People with Medicare,* and *Medicare and Managed Care Plans.*

Understanding the costs, scope, and limits of Medicare is quite important. You will learn, for example that once parents are eligible, participation in the basic plan (Part A, Hospital Insurance), costs them nothing. Instead participation is financed through the Social Security (FICA) tax paid by workers and their employers. Parents may be entitled to Part A benefits under either the Social Security or Railroad Retirement system or certain government parallels, if they worked a sufficient period in federal, state, or local government to be insured.

HOSPITAL INSURANCE (PART A)

Part A offers a package of services. It helps pay for in-patient hospital stays, in-patient care in a skilled nursing facility or psychiatric hospital, and some home health and hospice care following a hospital stay. Covered services include blood transfusions, lab tests, X-rays, operating and recovery room costs, and rehabilitation services. To qualify for home health expenses, your parent must be "homebound" and "need" part-time or "intermittent" skilled nursing services (defined as care that can only be performed by, or under the supervision of licensed nursing personnel).

Terminally ill beneficiaries may also choose hospice care for symptom management and pain relief.

Medicare Part A (Hospital Benefits) pays full hospital bills (after the beneficiary pays a specified deductible) for the first sixty days of each hospitalization. This does not cover private-duty nursing or extra charges for private rooms. In 1983, to control the high costs of hospital care and discourage pro-longed hospital stays, Medicare instituted a formula for fixed-price reimbursements based on categories of particular medical conditions and the average length of hospital stay for them. These categories are known as "Diagnosis Related Groups" (DRGs). They cause considerable conflicts between hospitals and patients because the hospital is paid the same amount, whether a patient leaves earlier or later than the average stay. That creates an incentive for hospitals to discharge patients rapidly—sometimes too rapidly—in order to save money on reimbursements. This means that sick people may no longer be allowed to recuperate in the hospital.

To protect patients, Congress created a national network of Medicare Peer Review Organizations (PROs) which review hospital decisions and discourage premature patient discharges. Unfortunately, most families do not know Medicare rules or understand these procedures to safeguard patients. But you need to know the rules so you can act as an advocate if told that a hospital discharge is imminent, and you do not agree. If you know that your parent is entitled to a review of that decision, and to continued Medicare coverage during the interim, you can learn the steps to follow should you wish to appeal. These steps are detailed in *Your Medicare Handbook,* published by the Health Care Financing Administration and it is available free. In fact, some hospitals have "patient advocates" on staff to provide this appeal service.

Because Medicare Part A provides some nursing home care after a hospital stay, most people believe long-term care needs are also covered. But Medicare pays for less than 1 percent of all nursing home costs. This is because Medicare focuses on acute rather than chronic care. Moreover, for acute cases it only covers care in skilled nursing facilities for a maximum of 100 days. Even then, patients in 1995 were required to pay $89.50 each day after the twentieth day of confinement.

In addition, while Medicare covers "intermittent" care at home, it does not cover full-time nursing care at home; or drugs; or home-delivered meals; or homemaker or chore services; or blood transfusions; or custodial or any personal care services such as help with bathing, eating, or dressing.

In short, Medicare draws a sharp line between medical crises or acute illnesses, and long-term care services for chronic conditions. The first group is covered. The other is not. Yet costs of managing disabling chronic conditions which require custodial care are faced by nearly half the noninstitutionalized elderly.

MEDICAL INSURANCE, PART B

Part B, Medical Insurance, is an optional, voluntary program with a monthly charge. Part B helps pay for doctor visits (whether received at home, a doctor's office, a clinic, a nursing home, or a hospital). It also helps pay for tests and outpatient hospital services. Retirees are automatically enrolled in Part B when they become eligible for Part A, unless they state otherwise. The monthly premiums are then deducted from their Social Security checks.

Medicare Part B pays 80 percent of "approved charges" for covered doctor expenses after a $100 yearly deductible apart from the deductible for hospital costs. Part B will reimburse up to 80 percent of costs for certain medical assistance equipment such as wheelchairs, hospital beds, and grab bars for the shower. Part B *does not cover:* 50 percent of approved charges for out-patient mental health treatment; charges in excess of a maximum yearly limit for independent physical or occupational therapy; prescription drugs; dental care or dentures; routine physical examinations; cosmetic surgery; eye, foot care, or hearing loss examinations; care received outside the United States.

STEP 31—UNDERSTAND HOW PRIVATE HEALTH INSURANCE (MEDIGAP) POLICIES FILL SOME MEDICARE GAPS

Your parents do not have to be poor to be frightened by the prospect of catastrophic health costs. And they do not have to be poorly educated to be victimized by confusing information about insurance. Currently 95 percent of the nation's elderly are covered by Medicare Parts A and B. Two-thirds pay for one or more "Medicare supplements" (also known as "Medigap" insurance) sold by private insurance companies. Medigap policies are attractive because they plug several holes in Medicare coverage. They may include long hospital stays exceeding sixty days, the uncovered portion (20 percent) of doctors' bills and lab tests, and outpatient prescription drugs. But this list is limited.

If Medicare does not cover health costs, people believe their private supplemental insurance will. In fact, basic Medigap policies only supplement the co-payment portion of qualified Medicare payments. Co-payment refers to the portion of an otherwise-covered medical bill that the patient pays. Thus, Medigap only reimburses for costs covered by Medicare.

For example, since Medicare pays for inpatient hospital

stays based on the flat-rate "Diagnosis Related Groups" (DRGs), and since the hospital is paid a pre-set amount for each procedure, once the DRG has expired, private insurance will not cover continued hospitalization that is not "medically necessary." If neither Medicare nor private insurance pays for custodial care, these expenses are covered by "private pay." Which means a parent's pocket. Or yours.

In 1990 Congress passed a law to protect consumers purchasing Medigap insurance policies. These consumer protection laws guarantee that such policies are renewable, provide six months of open enrollment at age sixty-five, and eliminate waiting periods for replacement policies. They also prohibit high-pressure sales practices and simplify the number of available plans to ten standard Medicare supplement policies, specifying exactly what benefits each plan must contain. In addition, consumers have a thirty-day free look and are entitled to a full refund should they change their minds.

Although all ten plans may not be available in every state, the basic benefits available to all Medicare recipients include: co-payment coverage for hospital stays of 61–90 days and 91–150 days; coverage of up to 365 additional days per lifetime; a 20 percent co-payment of Medicare Part B's allowed amount (above the $100 annual deductible); and coverage for the first three pints of blood received per calendar year.

Consumers may choose bare-bones coverage with lower costs, or opt for fancier packages. For example, plan "J," the most comprehensive and expensive, also offers insurance for some preventive health care screening procedures, foreign travel emergencies, and prescription drugs. Plans "D," "G," "I," and "J" include some at-home personal care services covered by Medicare for patients receiving skilled home care following illness, injury, or surgery.

Since you may be the one who fills out the forms and files the claims, it is important to understand the scope and cost of various Medigap insurance options. There is great variation in price for the same coverage. You will want to compare price, service, and reliability. While gathering data, keep these pointers in mind:

- See whether your parents are already insured. They may not need Medigap insurance at all . . .

    IF they are enrolled in a prepayment plan, such as a Medicare Health Maintenance Organization (HMO), that contracts with Medicare;

    IF they are eligible for continued coverage under an employer-provided health insurance policy (See Step 32);

    IF they are low income and eligible for Medicaid (see Step 33); or,

    IF they are not eligible for Medicaid but fall below certain income levels and have limited assets. In this case, they may qualify for government support which pays their Medicare premiums and may provide supplemental coverage.

- Get help analyzing coverage, costs, and quality. Recent legislative changes in the Medicare program all point to a greater role for private health insurance, more available insurance options, and a greater need for consumer education. The good news is that help through the Medicare maze is available—for free! By federal law, every state has an insurance counseling program for seniors. These programs offer telephone and in-person counseling, printed materials, help in choosing coverage, and assistance in navigating the insurance claim or appeal process. For example, the Pennsylvania program, Apprise, is part of the State Department of Aging. According to Denise Hussar, Chief of the Division of Health and Consumer Education,

CONSUMER BEWARE

Before buying or switching Medigap insurance, follow the "Buyer Beware" advice of the Health Care Financing Administration (HCFA), which administers Medicare:

Shop carefully before you buy.
Do not buy more policies than you need.
Consider alternatives.
Check for "preexisting condition" exclusions.
Beware of replacing existing coverage.
Be aware of maximum benefits
Know who you are dealing with. Keep agents' or companies' names, addresses, and telephone numbers.
Take your time choosing. Do not be pressured. Remember: Policies that supplement Medicare are neither sold, serviced, nor guaranteed by the federal government. State insurance departments approve policies sold by insurance companies; this means they only need to meet minimum provisions of state law.
If you decide to buy, complete the application carefully. Look for an outline of coverage.
Do not pay in cash.

Finally, should your parents select a policy and sign up, make sure policy delivery and premium refunds (if parents decide to cancel) are prompt.

in a typical sixty-day period in 1995, of 3,000 people counseled. Most sought help with Medicare benefits, information on Medigap policies, or help processing claims. Other inquiries focused on Medicaid benefits, long-term care issues, medicare disability, medication benefits, and coordinated care. (See Appendix 2 on p. 245)

STEP 32—CONSIDER ALTERNATIVES TO MEDIGAP INSURANCE: MEDICARE MANAGED CARE, PPOS, FEE-FOR-SERVICE, EMPLOYER GROUP INSURANCE

The Budget Reconciliation Bill passed by Congress but vetoed by President Clinton in early 1996 included major changes to contain, if not reduce, the burgeoning costs of the Medicare. The bill's "Medicare-Plus" program expanded the range of Medicare options for eligible seniors, using not only the current "Fee-For-Service" (FFS) option, but fostering greater use of "managed-care" programs offered by Medicare health maintenance organizations (HMOs) or preferred provider organizations (PPOs).

Under fee-for-service (FFS), the patient selects the doctor or hospital for service. The third party insurer (Medicare) pays most of the bill. So long as the providers are Medicare-approved and the services are covered by Medicare, there are practically no restrictions on consumer choice of doctor, hospital, procedures, or medical tests. Critics feel the FFS system increases Medicare expenditures because it has no limit and encourages unnecessary tests and procedures. HMOs instead emphasize preventive medicine, and coordination of care.

Preferred Provider Organizations (PPO)

In this variation of managed care more closely related to fee-for-service, a group of practitioners contract with employers, unions or third-party administrators to provide health services at competitive rates. Employees are free to choose among the physicians. They can use their regular doctor, even if he or she does not participate in the PPO. In this case, they usually pay a higher co-payment fee. PPOs, like HMOs use primary care physicians to assure hospitalizations occur only when necessary.

Managed Care

"Managed care" is a new buzzword in healthcare. Unlike Medigap policies described in Step 31, managed-care plans usually demand only small payments by clients for each medical visit, rather than large deductibles.

Medicare
A health maintenance organization (HMO) is an example of a managed-care plan. An HMO provides health care to enrolled members for a flat monthly fee. Doctors and other providers are paid a salary or are under contract. Often the medical facilities are owned by the HMO. Most HMOs provide eye and ear exams, dental care, and prescription drugs at little or no cost. They also feature services such as diet and exercise advice, or even health club memberships. BUT your parents have to live in the HMO territory to receive services. Members are also locked in to care provided within the particular HMO network. Enrollees who travel outside that territory or seek care from nonparticipating providers usu-

ally find, to their distress, that they are only covered for emergency or urgently needed care.

Medicare managed-care plans vary in terms of where services are provided, the amount of care, how much government pays, whether they are for-profit or non-profit, the degree of patient choice, and the types of covered services. According to an HMO marketing representative quoted in *US News & World Report* (June 1995), the main advantage of HMOs is what they *don't* do:

> They don't take as large a bite out of members' budgets, nor do they require hassling with claim forms. HMO enrollees continue to pay Medicare their monthly $46.10 Part B premium for physician and outpatient care, but many Medicare HMOs charge no additional premium. They collect a flat monthly fee per member from Medicare, regardless of how much care is given. . . . HMOs impose no deductible and, at most, only a $10 co-payment for each physician visit.

The theory is that healthcare costs are contained under managed care programs because access to care is filtered through the primary care doctor, who acts as a gatekeeper. According to an HMO manager, "patients do what their doctors tell them to do; therefore if you tell doctors how to practice medicine, you can cut costs."* To make managed care more attractive for Medicare beneficiaries, lawmakers want to ease restrictions and allow Medicare members to go "outside" their plan for other needed services, as long as they pay

*Wall Street Journal, May 2, 1995.

additional charges for this option. This new form of Medicare managed care is called Point-of-Service (POS). However, even with this option, should your parent need expensive or complicated surgery, the final choice of doctor or hospital may be based on the cost to the HMO, not the quality or experience of either physician or medical facility.

Nearly three million Medicare beneficiaries—almost 10 percent of total enrollees—have joined Medicare "managed-care" organizations instead of regular Medicare programs. In 1994 alone, the number of people in the most common type of Medicare HMO rose 27 percent. The number of approved HMO plans jumped to 154 from 109.

The following section offers consumer tips on questions to ask before signing on to *any* HMO. To learn more, call the Medicare Hotline (1-800-638-6833) to order such valuable pamphlets as *Your Medicare Handbook,* and *Medicare and Managed Care Plans.* You can also call the state Health Insurance Counseling office to ask for the names of approved Medicare HMOs in your parents area (see p. 245).

CONSUMER BEWARE

Under present rules, Medicare beneficiaries can opt out of Medigap or switch *into* HMOs at any time. However, should your parents try an HMO and decide they do not like its restrictions, they may have trouble renewing their old fee-for-service Medigap policy. This is especially true if they have been diagnosed with a new condition in the interim. Should they decide to test the HMO waters, consumer advocates recommend keeping a Medigap policy for a while to make sure the new plan is satisfactory.

CONSUMER BEWARE

HMOs are not for everyone. Managed care may look attractive to *younger and healthier* retirees because of low rates, but it may severely limit choice, access, and quality of care for more frail members.

According to HCFA, 10 percent of the sickest Medicare enrollees account for 70 percent of total Medicare expenditures. Critics worry that HMO insurers will "cherry-pick" members, selecting for enrollment only those in better health in order to increase their profits. Since HMOs are reimbursed on a monthly per-head basis for care, whether or not retirees seek care, plans with healthy members and strict limits to specialist care will make more profits than those with a less healthy membership pool.

When evaluating choice, you should compare benefits, costs, choices of medical providers, and other features. Unlike Medigap, there are no national standards for Medicare HMO plans. The most common consumer complaints are:

- refusal to pay for emergency room or urgent care (most frequent complaint).

- deceptive enrollments.

- illegal health screening as a prerequisite of membership.

- refusal to refer patients to specialists.

- failure to inform HMO members of their appeal rights.

- inadequate monitoring to document compliance with federal law.

- lack of public access to current data.

- failure to provide minimally mandated Medicare benefits for the seriously ill and disabled, especially for nursing home and home health care.*

*Source: United Seniors' *Special Report 40* on Medicare HMOs (Washington, D.C., September 1995. To order, call, 212-0393-6222).

Know Your Rights

Just as your parents have consumer protection rights against premature discharge from a hospital, they have rights to grievance and appeals procedures under a Medicare HMO. Plans are also required by federal law to inform members of these rights. But the five-step appeal process can take up to two years. When delays in treatment could be harmful to parents' health, their choice may be either to forego care or pay out of their pockets and then appeal for reimbursement. If HMO complaints arise, act promptly; get copies of all relevant information; and keep a paper trail with dates, names, what occurred, and what was said.

Shop Around

In shopping for an HMO, get as much help as you can. You might check to see if local consumer groups have ranked plans in your parents' area. For example, the *1995 Washington Consumer's Checkbook* review of Health Insurance for Medicare Recipients surveyed federal retirees participating in the Federal Employees Health Benefits HMOs. They asked participants to rate plans by such care criteria as access, quality, doctors, information, customer service, and coverage, as well as such practical care items as waiting time in doctor's office, coordination of care, results and choice of specialists. Or, you might search for information on the World Wide Web. The National Committee for Quality Assurance (NCQA), an independent not-for-profit organization assesses and rates managed-care plans nationwide, including Medicare HMOs. Its online site offers evaluations of the quality of individual HMOs accredited by the group, along with information on its evaluation criteria (see the Eldercare Internet address, p.133).

Employer Group Health Insurance

Your parents may still be working after sixty-five and wish to retain private health insurance through their own employer or the employer of their working spouse. Although the plans are not subject to Medigap policy regulations, advantages may include lower group rates, no waiting periods or exclusions for preexisting health conditions, and possible coverage for prescription drugs and routine dental work. If one parent works, and retains coverage with an employer group plan, that plan becomes the primary payer of claims. Medicare will be secondary. For more information, speak with a benefits counselor at Social Security or the working spouse's benefits department.

PLAN HOW TO PAY FOR LONG-TERM CARE

An estimated eight million older Americans experience illness, disability, or injury so severe they can no longer manage the tasks of daily living and need long-term care. According to the Administration on Aging, five million people with such conditions live at home assisted by some twelve million family caregivers, primarily women. Half of all caregivers also work outside the home.

What is "long-term care?"The phrase refers to a range of formal and informal services for the health, personal care, and social needs of people who have either chronic illness or a mental, that is, cognitive, or physical disability which make it difficult for them to care for themselves. They may need care at home, or round-the-clock attention in a special facility. Long-term care services are not provided only in a nursing home. They are available in assisted-living facilities, through community programs like adult day care, and home healthcare or home care. (As a rule of thumb, home healthcare refers to medical care to maintain health. Home care has to do with other personal needs.)

What are the chances your parents will require such care at all? It depends on their sex, health, age, family health history, and genetics, along with their style of life. And how likely is it they will need nursing home care? According to a 1991 report in the *New England Journal of Medicine,* 43 percent of all Americans reaching age sixty-five can expect to spend some time in a nursing home. One out of five will spend five years or more there.

If your parents retire at sixty-five, they will likely live another twenty years. The challenge is to stretch their income to meet needs for those two decades, and stretching will probably be necessary. Only 25 percent of the elderly and only 15 percent of those over eighty-five have annual incomes over $35,000. The median net assets of elderly women living alone are $12,500—barely enough to cover four months of nursing home care. Fifty-three percent of elderly married couples and 71 percent of elderly singles get half their monthly support from Social Security checks. This single income source and the average annual Social Security benefits were well under $10,000 at the end of 1994.

Thus, asset income becomes increasingly important with age. More specifically, careful management of assets to maximize their income is important.

Advance planning for potentially devastating long-term care is a must in today's society. The longer the lead time, the greater your family's choices, and the better the likely solutions.

- If your parents have limited resources, you can help them learn about available benefits from public programs like SSI, the Veterans' Administration, and Medicaid.

- If your parents have too much money to qualify for public programs, do not wish to spend it all on their own care, and want to reserve funds for their spouse or family, you can get them professional help to design a plan for meeting unexpected demands.

- If your parents want to be cared for at home, choose their own nursing care, and not totally depend on you for their financial and living support, you can help them evaluate long-term care insurance.

- Regardless of your parents' resources, you can help them stretch income from the non-Social Security part of the ledger. For example, one or both of your parents may delay retirement and continue working. They may rent out some space in their home (or garage). They might borrow against the equity of their home or even sell it, investing appreciated growth in income-producing assets. Steps 33, 34 and 35 will help you get acquainted with this unknown terrain.

STEP 33—INVESTIGATE BENEFITS FROM SSI, THE VETERANS ADMINISTRATION, AND MEDICAID FOR ASSISTANCE IN PAYING FOR LONG-TERM HOME OR NURSING HOME CARE

SSI

If your parents have monthly income below the poverty level (In 1996, the poverty level income was $470 per month for an individual, or $705 per month for a couple), *and* assets of less than $2,000 (individual) or $3,000 (couple), *and* are residents, U.S. citizens or lawfully admitted immigrants, they may be eligible for SSI, the Supplemental Security Income Program of Social Security. Begun in 1974, SSI provides federal monthly cash payments to the needy elderly, blind, and disabled. Many states supplement the Federal benefit to bring total benefits up to the poverty level. SSI also confers eligibility for other benefits like food stamps, home support programs, and Medicaid.

SSI is a much underused program. Only half the elderly persons who qualify for SSI actually receive benefits. You might want to call the Social Security Administration (1-800-772-1213) to see if your parents qualify. If you schedule an appointment with a Social Security representative to help your parent(s) apply, bring the following documents: a Social Security card; birth certificate; information about your parents' home, such as a mortgage or lease; and bank books, insurance policies, or other information about assets and monthly income. If signing up for disability, also bring the names, addresses, and telephone numbers of your parents' doctors, hospitals, and clinics.

VA PENSIONS

Are you and your parents aware that many veterans, their dependents, and their survivors are eligible for benefits from the Department of Veterans Affairs, *even if the veteran does not have a service-connected disability?* Low-income vets and their survivors who qualify for a "needs-based pension" can obtain VA cash grants and help with healthcare costs.

This program may also help low-income parents pay for Medigap health insurance, prescription drugs, or home care. The monthly basic pension for a veteran is currently $669. For a surviving dependent it is $448. Those who qualify and are substantially confined to their home by one or more permanent disabilities may receive additional funds. There are further sums available for the blind, patients in nursing homes, or those needing help with such "activities of daily living" (ADL) as bathing, feeding, or dressing. Other veterans' programs may help pay for unreimbursed medical expenses. (Call the local office of the Veterans Administration for further information.)

MEDICAID

If your parents have limited financial resources and also meet state medical/disability requirements, or if they are in a nursing home, they may qualify for Medicaid.

Established under Title XIX of the Social Security Act in 1965 as companion legislation to Medicare, Medicaid is an entitlement program jointly funded and administered by federal and state governments. Federal law currently controls the basic structure of the state-administered programs.

Why does this matter to a middle-class caregiver? Because Medicaid is the resource of last resort to pay the costs of long-term care when those costs have depleted a family's financial reserves. Custodial nursing home care for the frail elderly is a huge expense, with average costs of $38,000 a year in 1995. Those costs can quickly consume even a large nest egg. Without Medicaid, once that nest egg has vanished, the nursing home might discharge your parent—or ask you to pay those costs.

Medicaid finances health and long-term care for the poor elderly, including "the medically needy" impoverished by long-term care costs. The program has two components. It helps pay for nursing home care, and it offers some relief for those who try to manage long-term care at home. In 1994 there were more than four million over-65 Medicaid recipients. This number included almost one and a half million persons living in nursing homes or intermediate care facilities. It also included half a million frail elderly who counted on Medicaid support for home health services.*

In that same year Medicaid paid for slightly over half of the total nursing home care in the United States almost $38 billion. Most of the remaining costs were paid by families out of savings and retirement income. Only a small percentage were covered by private long-term care insurance.

*Source: Medicaid Statistics Staff, Medicaid Bureau, Health Care Financing Administration (HCFA), March 28, 1996.

Medicaid Eligibility for the "Medically Needy" in Nursing Facilities

A nursing home resident's "medically needy" eligibility for Medicaid kicks in after he or she "spends down," that is, exhausts personal savings. This situation occurs for half of all nursing home residents within six months of entry.

Once a person is certified for Medicaid, most medical costs—either in a nursing home or at home—are covered. Your parents can qualify only if they meet strict Medicaid financial tests. These tests generally include limited assets and limited income, though there are wide variations in eligibility thresholds, benefits, services, and spending among the fifty states. Under the general rules, *exempted assets* include the value of a home, car, household goods, personal items, and funeral costs or burial plots. *Countable assets* include everything else: IRAs, stocks, bonds, and savings.

Both Medicare and Medicaid help older people finance medical and health expenses. But these programs leave wide, discriminatory gaps between coverage for acute and chronic long-term care.

This fact was dramatized in 1995 testimony of Janet L. Kuhn, an expert in Virginia's eldercare law before a Virginia Women Attorneys' Association Board of Directors hearing.

Milton Millionaire can run up hundreds of thousand of dollars in hospital medical bills for a heart condition involving by-pass surgery and time in and out of the Intensive Care Unit. ALL of his medical bills will be covered by a combination of Medi*care* and Medi*gap* supplemental insurance. Medicare is available to everyone eligible for social security; eligibility is not "means tested"—i.e., eligibility for benefits is not related to income or assets. . . .

Joe Doe, a retired plumber, $80,000 house with no mortgage, one old car, a "nest egg" of $75,000 or so and a family retirement income of about $30,000 per year, including his wife's $300 a month Social Security check would receive the same Medicare benefits as Milton—but if poor Joe has the bad luck to develop Alzheimer's disease instead of a heart condition, the same several hundred thousand dollars worth of medical benefits would not be there for him.

Moral: Unless you're a millionaire, pick your illness carefully. No matter how long a devoted spouse or adult child manages to care for an Alzheimer's patient at home . . . nursing home care will eventually be required.

To sum up, your parents can become eligible for Medicaid in any of three ways: *First,* if they qualify for cash assistance under the federal Social Security Supplemental Security Income program (SSI) (see p. 168); *second,* by a "spend down" in which healthcare service costs exceed income and assets, creating "impoverishment"; *third,* through a supplementary healthcare insurance program—for Medicare recipients not poor enough to qualify for Medicaid—but whose incomes fall under the official federal poverty level.

Medicaid Support for Home Care

Not all Medicaid beneficiaries live in nursing homes. Increasingly they live in the community. Medicaid now underwrites almost one-fourth of all home health spending in the United States. This includes *skilled home healthcare* (in all states) and through home and community-based waivers, *personal care* (in 29 states). Medicaid home health expenditures include costs for part-time skilled nursing, homemaker home health services, and medical supplies and equipment—for those eligible. Home care coverage may also include reimbursement for adult day care programs and some relief time ("respite care") for caregivers.

New York's Nursing Home Without Walls (NHWW) program is one example. NHWW began in 1979 to provide long-term care custom-tailored to individual needs. Eligible participants receive a periodic comprehensive health, social, and environmental assessment which covers family status and informal support networks as well as the participant's own care requirements.

The NHWW Medicaid services in New York include the normal therapies, nutrition counseling, and audiology. But they also include medical supplies and equipment, personal care, home health aides, homemakers, housekeepers, social day care, respite care, home-delivered meals, group meals, transportation, housing improvement, home maintenance, personal emergency response systems, and moving assistance. A social worker coordinates the services needed, provides counseling, and keeps in touch.

Contact your parents local Department of Human Services or Area Agency on Aging to learn about eligibility (see also Step 34, p. 177).

MEDICAID PROTECTIONS FOR FAMILIES

Over the past three decades, Congress has enacted protective laws which recognize how long-term care in a nursing home can drain a family's resources. A 1995 fact sheet on federal Medicaid policy prepared by the Los Angeles office of the National Senior Citizens Law Center sets out these national protections. They include:

1. **Guaranteed Eligibility**

   Under current federal law, the elderly or disabled who need nursing home care but do not have the funds to pay the full private care rate are entitled to have Medicaid pay the bill after the individual assigns most of his or her income to the facility.

2. **Protection Against Discrimination**

   A nursing home resident cannot be discharged from a certified facility when he or she runs out of money and applies for Medicaid. Family members do not have to impoverish themselves to continue paying the bill after the resident has exhausted his or her private funds.

3. **Protection Against Supplementation**

   Nursing facilities are prohibited from seeking payments above the "Medicaid rate" from spouses and other family members. The Medicaid rate must be accepted as payment in full.

4. **Protection Against Filial Responsibility**

   Adult children of nursing home residents are not legally responsible to pay for their parent's care.

5. **Protection Against Estate Recovery**

   The state cannot recover the Medicaid costs from a beneficiary's estate during the lifetime of the Medicaid beneficiary, or the lifetime of a spouse or dependent or disabled children.

6. **Protection of Planning for Disabled Children**
   Individuals may transfer assets to a trust for a disabled child without losing Medicaid eligibility.

7. **Protection of Income, Resources, and Shelter for the "Community Spouse"**
   Should your father need to go to a nursing home, how much money from his pensions and benefits can go to his wife, if she does not have enough income on her own?

   To deal with this problem of "spousal impoverishment," the Medicare Catastrophic Coverage Act of 1988 provided a basic living allowance to support the spouse-at-home. Before President Reagan signed this law, community spouses in most states could receive no more than $340 per month from their institutionalized spouse, even if they had no income themselves. By 1995, the "minimum maintenance needs allowance" was $1,254, plus excess shelter adjustments of up to $1,871 monthly.

8. **Protection of the Homestead for Remaining Family Members**
   The state cannot place a lien on the homestead while it is lived in by dependent or disabled children—or by children who have cared for their parents for a fixed period of time. The state cannot seize a homestead in the estate of a deceased Medicaid beneficiary as long as dependent or disabled children live there.

Twenty years ago, federal Medicaid law had only minimal protections for families of nursing home residents. But one of the most important was a prohibition against nursing homes demanding "supplementation" of the Medicaid rate. When Medicaid costs started to skyrocket in the early 1980s, Congress gave states greater authority to recover state costs for long-term care through liens on real estate and "estate recovery." But Congress was clear that such cost recovery could only be pursued when the home was not needed for use by a spouse, a dependent, or disabled children. In 1993 Congress tightened the noose and *required* states to undertake "estate recovery" of Medicaid expenditures, although not the cost of liens.

Under the 1995 GOP budget plan, vetoed by President Clinton in 1996, Medicaid as an entitlement program would have been repealed and replaced by a block grant program called "Medigrant," administered by the states. The program retained current protections against spousal impoverishment. It retained federal nursing home standards, but gave responsibility for enforcing them to the states. Federal authorities would still be able to inspect nursing homes and levy fines for inadequate care, if a state failed to do so. The states would have reported compliance and provided information to consumers about the standards.

With the shift of authority and program responsibility to the states, all eight federal Medicaid provisions "preempting" state laws would also have been repealed. State Medicaid cost-cutting provisions which have long been blocked by federal rules would suddenly have come to life. Those provisions typically require adult children to pay for the care of their parents, permit "supplementation," and allow states to place liens on family homes in which the spouse and other dependent family members live. They do not offer protection from discrimination in admission to and transfer and discharge from nursing homes if the prospective or current resident has exhausted his or her resources and does not have enough monthly income to pay the full nursing home bill.

In short, block grants for Medicaid could eliminate basic protections for the frailest of society's members and their caregivers. Current proposals to reduce a growing rate of long-term care expenditures through cuts in eligibility, services, and standards are quite discouraging for families needing extensive long-term care.

STEP 34—SEEK PROFESSIONAL HELP TO PREPARE A LONG-TERM CARE STRATEGY

Healthcare and benefit regulations, even if they don't change, are already very complex.

The rules for "what counts" and "what doesn't" establishing eligibility for SSI, VA pensions, and Medicaid come straight out of *Alice in Wonderland.* For example, Social Security is considered income for VA pension purposes. But VA benefits do not affect Social Security benefits. SSI is excluded in determining eligibility for (and the amount of) VA pensions. But your basic VA pension is considered income for SSI purposes.

If your parents' costs outstrip their ability to pay, you will need to explore financial support from all sources—including these public benefits. From one point of view, your parents worked all their lives and paid taxes to be able to rely on help in time of need. Accepting them is not taking charity, any more than is accepting a private pension. Even if your parents feel differently and choose not to apply for these programs, as consumers you should know what they are and what they can do for informed decision making.

State laws vary. So using the Medicaid safety net for the "medically needy" facing catastrophic costs requires help from an expert familiar with the rules where your parents reside. If you have prepared the checklists of Steps 1–21, you already have a handle on your parents' needs, their financial picture, and the support they currently receive. To learn more about their eligibility for federal benefits, visit or call a benefits counselor at the Social Security Administration or the Area Agency on Aging in your parents' community. Better yet, contact the family attorney, local Bar Association, or area Legal Counsel for the Elderly to find an expert in "Elder Law"—and arrange a consultation. You may find you need several consultations. So don't forget to ask what documents you should bring to that first appointment. You will save time and money because the expert will be able to focus faster on planning to prevent the "worst case" from coming true.

How can you protect your parents (and yourselves)? By using information based on current law and advance legal and financial planning. Here are some planning measures your parents might consider:

· Divide or Transfer Jointly-owned Assets
  Many people are now familiar with estate planning to reduce taxes if a parent dies. Similar steps to divide or shift income may be important to assure eligibility for long-term care. When you helped prepare your parents' financial records, you noted which of their assets were held

separately or jointly. Shifting those assets can have important effects on eligibility for Medicaid or other financial assistance programs. But it can also have serious tax consequences, so be careful to consult a lawyer or financial planner before you act. Similarly, transferring property between spouses (or between parents and children) *must* be done at appropriate times and in appropriate ways to meet strict, constantly changing federal and state laws.

· Protect Exempt Assets

Medicaid regulations generally allow participants to keep one major asset—their home. They also exclude that home from eligibility and payment considerations so long as your parents, their caretaker, or a dependent relative lives there. But some states (like California) allow a lien to be imposed on the house if its Medi-Cal beneficiary "cannot reasonably be expected to return home"—for example, or has been in an institution for over six months and has no discharge plan. You must consult an attorney to learn about ways of protecting exempt assets like the family home. The rules are different in each state.

· Make Gifts

Kaufman and Hart taught us *You Can't Take It With You.* But your parents can't even give it away as they wish. Whether making gifts to their children or grandchildren or the neighbor next door, assets must be gifted several years before anticipation of death or eligibility for programs like Medicaid. Gifting may make perfect legal sense for the poor or middle class as well as the wealthy. It may also please the giver and receiver. But your parents need to be comfortable with the option. Don't be surprised if they are not in the Santa Claus mode. Concern about outlasting their money may prompt them to hang onto every penny, and they may be right to do so.

STEP 35—CONSIDER LONG-TERM CARE INSURANCE TO HELP FINANCE EXTENDED CARE

Given the current budget climate, you should not count on government programs to cover increasingly expensive long-term care for our nation's elderly. So if your parents have potentially disabling conditions; have a net worth of at least $100,000; will not qualify for Medicaid (because they are too affluent) or Medicare nursing home care (because they probably will not have an illness or injury that requires moving from a hospital to a nursing home for sub-acute care), they should carefully consider long-term care insurance as a form of self-protection.

The need for this insurance can be measured by calculating how much present-day premiums protect against future out-of-pocket loss. Therefore before purchasing, you need to figure out how much you would have to invest to produce the same payment benefits through other financial means. Remember that risk varies with age and sex. Women live longer than men and use nursing homes more frequently. For the more affluent who may never qualify for Medicaid, but still want some protection, it is an option worth exploring.

Long-term care insurance differs from Medicare supplemental insurance. It focuses on intermediate and custodial care rather than short-term care for acute or sub-acute conditions. It can help your parent stay in a nursing home or other approved facility as a private-pay resident, if benefits like Medicare have run out. It can help your parent stay at home and participate in a community-care program.

By 1995 more than three and a half million persons had purchased such policies from over 150 companies. That compares to 200,000 policy holders and 40 companies in 1986. Yet these numbers are still relatively modest. Only 5 percent of the nation's elderly are covered. Why? Generally because the premiums are too expensive for those already over sixty-five or because seniors cannot qualify for the insurance due to pre-existing conditions or disabilities.

You may think your parents do not need another insurance policy because you will take care of them. While your sentiment is admirable, think twice. Consumer ignorance of the limits of Medicare and Medigap policies stiffens natural resistance to yet another insurance policy. But underestimating the need for coverage is risky. Medicaid and Medicare together may account for more than 60 percent of the nation's nursing home bill. But that still leaves 40 percent of $75 billion coming out of the pockets of patients and their families each year. The *average* 1995 yearly bill for a nursing home may be $38,000, according to *Consumer Reports* (September 1995). Yet a one-year stay can exceed $70,000. Moreover, since 1987, nursing home costs have been increasing at 10 percent a year.*

Long-term care insurance is expensive. Annual premiums average $1,500 when policies are purchased at age sixty-five, but can reach several thousand dollars if insurance is first pur-

*Partnership for Health Insurance Counseling, *Training Manual*, 1995.

chased ten years later. The longer one waits to buy, the higher the price.

Most long-term nursing home residents need custodial care—not Medicare-covered skilled nursing care. Such custodial care costs $60–100 per day. Similar care at home costs $150–300 per day for round-the-clock assistance.

Thus, long-term care insurance may be a good value, since its apparently expensive premiums can return much more in benefits. Benefits can include a daily payment of between $50 and $200 to defray custodial care expenses. Those daily payments may last several years, or as long as the policyholder lives. Several types of payment policies are currently available:

- Indemnity plans pay a fixed amount per day, regardless of what expenses are incurred or what another plan is paying.

- Actual cost plans pay out-of-pocket costs up to a daily maximum.

- Co-insurance plans pay a percentage of actual costs.

- Lump sum policies usually establish a sum to be used for covered services, which often include a daily limit.

When investigating this option, it is a good idea to contact the Senior Insurance counseling service in your parents state for more details as well as a representative from any company (See Appendix 2, p. 245). The insurance is complicated, and covers many options.

Insurers divide long-term care insurance into four main categories: skilled, intermediate, custodial, and services rendered in the home. Precise definitions vary between states and policies, and may turn out to be quite restrictive when applied. But any policy you consider should cover *all four* types of care. In addition you might ask if other community-based programs such as adult day care are covered.

Skilled care is medically necessary care continuously provided by a licensed medical professional under the supervision of a doctor. Restoring the patient to a condition approximating the state before illness or accident is the goal.

Intermediate care also requires medical supervision and skilled nursing. However, care is needed intermittently rather than continuously, over a prescribed period.

Custodial care primarily meets personal needs rather than medical needs. It includes help walking, getting out of bed, eating, and taking medicine. Such care could be provided by persons without professional training. But even if given by a professional in a skilled nursing facility, it is still considered custodial care.

Home healthcare is a mix of all the above. Its distinction is that it is provided in the home or community-based program rather than an institution. It covers companion and chore services as well as the professional services of a chemotherapist, occupational therapist, or lab.

Policies to consider should cover both a specified stay in a long-term care facility and certain home care services. The home care benefit may vary from 100 percent of the nursing home benefit (if medical or skilled care is needed) to half the nursing home benefit (if nonskilled services are required).

Virtually all long-term care insurance plans have "gate-keepers"—restrictions to determine eligibility for insurance reimbursement. Eligibility is generally based on the need for ongoing assistance for routine activities. Under some plans,

> CONSUMER BEWARE
>
> Long-term care insurance is confusing. Like Medigap insurance, it is difficult to compare policies and prices and easy to misread restrictions which may exclude those who need coverage most. Long-term care insurance is not a highly regulated industry. State regulators use minimum industry guidelines to protect consumers. But the guidelines remain and are bare minimums.
>
> As a result, there is no uniformity in the quality of coverage across the country. Comparisons between policies are difficult, and serious questions remain about coverage for care provided in sub-acute locations such as assisted-living facilities. The tips below identify potential pitfalls to look for before purchasing a long-term care insurance policy.
>
> • Clauses barring coverage of an individual without prior hospitalization, for pre-existing conditions, and for Alzheimer's disease.
>
> • Benefit rejection rates for those defined as poor health risks. Rejection may come during policy application. But it may come years later, when parents apply for benefits.

policy holders can qualify if they fail to meet certain tests measuring mental function. Some insurers specify functional need. Others leave more room for interpretation. Some policies require a physician certificate as well as a functional assessment. Some plans restrict the type of care facility or care provider. Others use case managers to determine if benefits will be paid. The case manager might work for an Area Agency on Aging, a government organization, the insurance company, or the providing home healthcare agency.

For a beneficiary to collect payment under long-term care insurance, companies insist that the "provider" of long-term care services—be it a *facility* (nursing home, assisted-living facility, continuing-care retirement community, hospice); a designated *agency* (home healthcare, adult day care center); or an *individual* (therapist, social worker, chore worker) must meet certain tests. Those tests include state licensing, Medicare certification, or listing by approved bodies.

Additional items to check are:

· Contract Information
Premiums. What is the annual cost? As with life insurance, generally the younger your parents are when they sign up, the lower the yearly cost.
Waiver of premiums. This option protects your parents from continued payment of premiums once coverage begins.
Terms of renewability. Policies must be "guaranteed renewable." Anything else means coverage may be cut off when benefits start to be needed.

· Admission and Eligibility Requirements
Type of facility covered. (See p. 218 for housing options.)
Length of waiting period. Some policies reimburse from the first day of long-term care. Others wait as long as 100 days. According to *Money* magazine, it is inadvisable to wait three months for benefits to start, because the median stay for most people who leave a nursing home alive is only sixty days.

· Limitations, Restrictions, and Exclusions
Restrictions for mental disorders. Do not buy a policy that excludes mental or nervous disorders such as Alzheimer's

disease. Nearly half of all nursing home residents are there because of loss of some mental faculties.

Exclusions for pre-existing conditions. Waiting periods before benefits start for medical conditions diagnosed or treated before policy purchase can range from ninety days to one year. But in some cases insurance with no exclusions can be purchased at higher premiums.

· Benefits

Coverage of skilled, intermediate, custodial, and home care. A plan that does not cover all levels of care is of little value. Learn how the company determines which level of care is needed and what kind of medical documentation you may need to initiate a claim. Many policies that cover home care may only cover home custodial services for a brief period. Try to make sure (before you purchase) that the policy covers the kinds of providers likely to be needed and for a realistic period of time. Different policies measure impairment using different scales of measurement and different definitions of impairment—for example, between those required for "home health care" and "home" care, and the types of eligible service providers who can perform for such care.

Daily benefits. Since indemnity policies pay a fixed amount, find one that adjusts benefits for inflation.

Length of coverage. The longer the benefit period the more desirable the policy. The average nursing home stay for custodial care residents is 2.4 years. On the other hand, skilled nursing care rarely extends six months. Should your parents choose to "age in place," that is, stay in their own homes, their need for home care can last years.

· Ratings
Purchase insurance only from companies with high financial ratings (A or A+), because the company needs to be
around long enough to pay. Several services rate insurance
companies for reserves, financial management, and similar factors. Your financial advisor or librarian can advise you
on where to find the ratings of the various firms.

When evaluating insurance plans and comparing benefit
restrictions, it is a good idea to seek help from a neutral insurance counseling program and follow up with some library
research. The AARP and the Health Insurance Association of
America both of Washington, D.C. have free booklets available upon request (see Appendix 4, p. 255).

ENSURE DECISION-MAKING AUTHORITY IN THE EVENT OF INCAPACITY

Planning for long-term care expenses helps mitigate financial disaster. Parents also need to decide on their preferences of healthcare choices and specify them through
written or video directives. This avoids other crises should
physical or mental incapacity cause a parent to lose decision-
making ability momentarily or permanently. In today's tech-
nological climate, written healthcare instructions—known
as advance directives—may protect parents' right to decide
their own medical treatment. They address not only use of
life support systems, but whether to start invasive medical
tests or insert feeding tubes. Advance directives can instruct

caregivers to use all medical technology available or to stop various medical interventions at a specific time.

Most of us do not plan for these end-of-life events and hate mentioning them. But contingency planning for devastating illness can relieve parents or family members of physical or mental suffering and heavy moral burdens. It can also give parents more assurance that their wishes will be carried out in the event they cannot do so.

What is meant by "incapacity" with respect to healthcare? A person is presumed capable to make treatment choices unless the attending doctor(s)—or a doctor plus proxy—determine that person either does not "understand or appreciate the nature and consequences of healthcare decisions, including benefits and risks of alternatives to any proposed healthcare decisions," or cannot communicate those preferences.

While your parents still manage their affairs, know what they want, and can speak their minds, do yourselves a favor and sit down to discuss how they would want you to act in worst-case scenarios. This is a discussion in which they may change their minds over time, given their age and their particular convictions as well as their health condition. It is also a discussion that benefits from very specific cases such as:

- whether they want cardiopulmonary resuscitation (CPR) which attempts to restore breathing if their heart should stop;

- whether they want any form of feeding tubes (inserted through their nose/throat), or other invasive forms of nutrition or hydration;

- whether they want intravenous (IV) therapy which provides water and medication through a tube in the vein;

- whether they should be placed on mechanical respirators if they cannot breathe on their own; and

- whether they want dialysis to clean their blood when their kidneys are no longer working, or antibiotics, or any form of surgery or invasive diagnostic tests in such circumstances.

These questions need discussing to let your parents personal values dictate their care. You all need to realize that their health may deteriorate suddenly and that most hospitals and even emergency rescue services will use all technology available to keep them physically alive, whether or not they are mentally incapacitated. If parents face a terminal illness or years in a coma, they may choose one set of options. If they have a treatable condition, they may choose another set.

As awkward as this conversation may be, you will not regret having it. Chances are your parents may already have thought about these issues but were reluctant to raise them with you. Chances are also good that they have not shared their views with their primary care physician. And chances are very great that they have not put their choices in writing—let alone executed a legally-effective advance directive.

Despite educational campaigns and federal laws supporting their use, more than two-thirds of Americans do not have advance directives in place. Indeed, according to the results of a 1995 American Medical Association survey, more than 62 percent of adults know almost nothing about them. The American Medical Association (AMA), the American

Association of Retired Persons (AARP), and the American Bar Association (ABA) have jointly co-authored a guide combining two key advance directives—the living will and the healthcare power of attorney. In these documents your parent would appoint a person to make healthcare decisions in event of incapacity, list the agent's powers, give instructions on end-of-life treatment, and record specific wishes regarding such topics as organ donation. They call for a signature by witnesses who know the individual but are not physicians, insurers, relatives, or estate beneficiaries for the individual. For a copy, send $2.00 and your request for *Shape Your Health Care Future* (D15803) to AARP Fulfillment (EE0940), 601 E St. NW, Washington, D.C. 20049.

After discussing these documents, and after they are signed (and notarized, if necessary), ask your parents to put cards in their wallets stating they have advance directives (See Appendix 4). You should also send a copy to their primary physician, and a copy to anyone who might be notified in an emergency. And bring a copy with you to the hospital, if a parent is admitted. The depressing fact is that even after you do all this planning, you may have to fight like a tiger to get some hospital or emergency team rescue squad to pay attention and honor your parents wishes.

STEP 36—DELEGATE AUTHORITY

Not all emergencies relate to health. Your parents may be away but need to complete a transaction at home. An alternate signator for their checking account can save worry or aggravation. Your parents will also need stand-in assistance should illness or frailty cause loss of ability to handle personal and business affairs. Parents may or may not realize this. But someone will have to manage their affairs, if they cannot.

Your parents may not want you to have authority to actually *perform* these tasks, but authority can be assigned or delegated to a family lawyer, an accountant, a friend, a relative, or the trust officer at a local bank. Here are some simple types of delegations:

- Authorization. Authority for a single purpose, such as access to a safe deposit box or bank account. This can usually be established at the bank through a simple form signed by you and your parents.

- Power of Attorney. A legal document which gives a named person (usually a spouse, relative, or friend) the power to act on behalf of another. Normally the person granting a power of attorney must be competent. That means the person must have the capacity to understand the nature and significance of the act not only at the time the power is signed but also when the designated attorney acts for the person. Thus an ordinary power of attorney is useless for dealing with disability, because the law normally requires *ongoing capacity* for the agent's actions to be valid. Therefore the power of attorney is void when the person granting it becomes incapacitated.

- Durable Power of Attorney lets your parent exercise full control over his or her affairs until incapacity occurs. But *after* incapacity, a durable power of attorney lets a trusted agent legally act for the parent. Thus the designated person can gain access to your parents' assets so bills are paid, checks are deposited, and affairs managed. Your parents should select their own agent for *both* healthcare and property issues. It is much better than being forced into the humiliating position of relying on the judgment of a court to make that selection in a public guardianship proceeding which declares the parent's incapacity. A durable power of attorney avoids the delays and costs of court proceedings. It can also be useful for tax, estate, and even Medicaid planning. For example, it can be used to save the family home should one spouse be incapacitated.

Durable power of attorney is a legal matter that *must* be pursued through an attorney. The parent must be protected from loss of control over his or her affairs and must fully understand the powers given to the agent(s) selected.

Finally, everyone involved should understand that such powers can only be used if or when the parent becomes incapacitated or disabled. They do not operate—and cannot be used to steal assets or thwart a parent's wishes when that parent is functioning. Until the parent is incapacitated, they may be revoked at any time. Even after they start operating, powers may be written to disappear after a specific period, or end with the death of the parent.

· Healthcare advance directive is the current buzzword for the document described at the beginning of this section. Your parents need this document to give instructions about their medical care if, in the future, they are incapacitated and cannot speak for themselves. The advance directive combines and expands two other documents—a living will which records parents' wishes about life support mechanisms or heroic measures, and a health care power of attorney which gives authority for the proxy to interpret the patient's instructions and make decisions. Unlike a living will, a healthcare power of attorney *is not limited to terminal illness.* (See Appendix 5, p. 260.)

· Representative Payee is a person who has authority to receive, sign, and cash another person's public benefit check, and is therefore responsible to help that person manage his or her finances. Persons who have a mental or physical disability, or a drug or alcohol problem, may need such help. Social Security *requires* a representative payee for persons on SSI due to drug or alcohol problems.

Social Security (or whatever agency administers the particular benefit) must authorize the representative payee arrangement. In turn, the representative payee must make an accounting to Social Security upon request of how the money has been used (usually annually). The representative payee can be removed for misconduct or if the person claims that the payee is no longer needed.

· Revocable living trusts also allow others to manage parents' property during incapacity. This legal instrument may be especially useful for more affluent elderly people to assure their "wishes for personal care and asset management can be implemented without court intervention." Virginia elder law attorney Janet Kuhn prefers this tool to protect her clients' control over their finances and care.

Kuhn recommends that where an affluent client has no immediate "successor trustee," the trust should authorize hiring of a geriatric care manager in event of incapacity. The trust can also specify a preference for care at home— even if the cost is greater than the cost of a nursing home—to insure that the care of the client takes precedence over the trustee's fiduciary duty to preserve assets. Should there be later incapacity, trustees have authority to manage property and make financial decisions on his or her behalf.

But again, seek professional advice. There are costs in setting up the trust, transferring assets to it, and managing its possessions.

- Joint tenancy with right of survivorship is the most common form on bank accounts, brokerage accounts, and other forms of property. It is known as "the poor person's will" because it automatically transfers assets to the surviving joint tenant. Under a joint tenancy either owner has equal access to and total control of all assets which are jointly held in both names. Often the two owners are spouses. However, problems may arise when one partner is incapacitated, financially irresponsible, or in a nursing home, and the remaining spouse wishes to sell or transfer assets. If a durable power of attorney exists or assets have previously been split, this problem disappears.

- Guardianship authorizes one individual to become a decision maker for another. Guardianships are controlled by state law. They may be limited or total, voluntary or involuntary, temporary or permanent. Delegated authority may be limited to guardians of the person (responsible for personal and healthcare decisions) or guardians of property (also called "conservators"). Guardianship can also cover both.

Creating a guardianship is time-consuming and costly.

Guardianship proceedings require filing of court petitions, notice to various parties, newspaper ads, and a trial involving presentation of expert medical evidence to prove the proposed ward suffers from some deficiency that makes him incapable of caring for himself or his property. Often that evidence will be opposed by a public defender or mental health advocate paid by the state to insure fair results.

In declaring a person incompetent and in need of a guardian, the court must find *first,* that the person suffers from a condition affecting his or her mental capacity; and *second,* that relevant functional disabilities result from this condition—for example, inability to do business, manage property, or make personal-care decisions. The consequences of this transfer of power to a guardian or conservator are drastic for the ward. The guardian, like a parent of a minor child, becomes responsible for the care, custody, and control of the ward. In many jurisdictions the ward may lose most adult rights, including rights to participate in business and professional activities, to vote, to drive, or to refuse (or consent to) medical treatment.

Each of these delegation procedures has limits which should be explained by experts. But some procedure of delegating responsibility and decision making may be critical when incapacity exists and parents require more extensive help over a period of time.

Dealing with these issues to guard against events that may never happen may be horrifying, tedious, expensive, and boring. But once you have worked through the insurance options, had your parents sign legal forms in case of incapacity, and developed plans to protect them if major illness or incapacity strikes you have removed a load of anxiety from your shoulders and theirs. In the process, you have probably added a thick stack to your parents' important documents and bought a filing cabinet to hold all the forms.

S E C T I O N   3

SECURING SAFETY AND WELFARE

The worst-case scenarios above may never happen. But sooner or later, you and your parents need to talk about housing and safety. The two may seem separate, but they are linked by your parents' ability—or lack of ability—to manage their lives independently. If your parents home is potentially hazardous, they will either have to improve its safety, or move to a more secure environment.

No matter where your parents live, you can help by:

· Checking and monitoring medications.

· Removing hazards.

· Making their home more comfortable.

· Getting them more help.

If your parents choose to move, they will need your help. Housing options range from:

· Finding a more manageable place where they can continue to live independently.

· Moving to a care facility.

· Moving in with you.

There is no easy formula for helping parents make these decisions—assuming they ask for help. The result depends on their mental, emotional, and physical conditions—and yours. But if they should ask, or you can suggest, here are hands-on things you can do:

STEP 37—CHECK MEDICATIONS

Medicines and age often do not mix—especially if an older person lives alone, is newly discharged from the hospital, or resides in a nursing home. Adverse drug reactions are a major problem for the elderly, particularly since many adverse reactions go undiagnosed. To secure the safety and welfare of those we love, the first step should be to check out their medications.

The Food and Drug Administration reports that over half of all Americans do not follow doctors' instructions for taking medicine. The 1989 report of the Inspector General of the U.S. Department of Health and Human Services found that two million seniors yearly are at risk for drug addiction due to regular prescriptions of tranquilizers or sleeping pills. It also found that in 1985 alone, adverse drug reactions were responsible for over a quarter-million hospitalizations, 32,000 hip fractures, 163,000 drug-induced mental impairments, and 61,000 cases of drug-induced Parkinsonism. Unsuspected drug effects can seriously impair the way older people function, feel, behave, and interact.

According to Martin Jinks, Chair of the Pharmacy Department at Washington State University, Americans over sixty-five take twice as much medication as the rest of us. Seventy-five percent take at least one prescription drug (and 92 percent take over the counter or prescription medication) regularly. Drug problems among the elderly are caused by multiple drug use, improper self-medication, and failure to follow instructions. For example, half the medicines are taken the wrong way because users cannot read or understand the label directions. Age also complicates how these medicines work when taken with other medications, or because older peoples' bodies absorb, metabolize, and excrete medicines differently than younger people.

Jinks recommends a professional drug assessment to evaluate the contents of medicines being taken, to eliminate all unnecessary drugs, to review dosage, and to assess the older person's ability to take prescribed medications. For example: Can Mom read the label? Does arthritis make it difficult for her to open and close the bottles or remove pills? Can she differentiate medicines by color? Can she take the right medicine in the right dose at the right time?

While good information on medicines is a key to preventing disaster, the best way to start is to put all medications (both prescription *and* over-the-counter) in a paper bag and take them to parents' local doctor or pharmacist. The Food and Drug Administration recently reported that 80 percent of Americans are reluctant to ask questions about the medicines they take. The pharmacist is an important player in your healthcare team, and should be consulted on the proper use of your parents' medicines.

You and your parents should know eight basic facts about each prescription drug they receive:

· The drug's correct name and what it is supposed to do.

· Exactly how and when to take the drug.

· How long to continue taking the drug.

· Precautions about concurrent use of alcohol, other drugs, or certain foods or activities.

· Side effects of the drug, and when to consult a doctor or pharmacist about them.

· What to do about missed doses.

· Shelf life of the drug, and any special storage requirements.

· Possible interactions with the other medications they are taking.

If your parents or you notice any adverse effects from their medicines, you should immediately notify their doctor.

REMOVE HAZARDS

For some parents, attachment to the old hearth is unimportant; costs, manageable space, and nearness to friends, family, or services are more critical. But for many older Americans, despite their home's growing inconvenience or isolation, the prospect of a move triggers paralyzing fears and anxieties.

Because your parents' home no longer fits their lifestyle does not mean they have to move, especially if they feel most secure staying put. You can support their desire to stay where they are—to "age in place"—by helping them make changes to their present home. That process is known as "retrofitting": removing obvious safety hazards, as well as improving comfort by making space and appliances easier for parents to use.

STEP 38—REMOVE HAZARDS AND MAKE HOME MORE COMFORTABLE

We know how dangerous homes can be for toddlers or young children. But homes are even more dangerous for older people who are not so resilient to falls, cuts, or burns. Weak eyes, hearing loss, muscle deterioration, or osteoporosis make the elderly more vulnerable to accidents and injuries.

Irma Dobkin, a Bethesda, Maryland interior designer/home improvement contractor, first became interested in disability design when she realized her luxurious home was totally inaccessible to her aging mother, who could not get out of the low-slung sofa or sunken tub. Recognizing that normal aging affects mobility, grip, and eyesight, Dobkin has developed a checklist for "aging in place" to prevent accidents and increase convenience. As cited in the *Washington Post* "Home Section" cover story, "Facing up to the Future" (November 2, 1995), her suggestions are both practical and inexpensive.

- Add lighting. Seniors require two to three times as much lighting as a twenty-year-old.

- Prevent scalding by setting water heaters at 120 degrees instead of the usual 150.

- Mount grab bars securely into wall studs to provide support in the shower and tub, or by a toilet.

- Install non-skid flooring, particularly in baths and kitchens.

- Replace loose rugs with low pile wall-to-wall carpeting.

- Choose sturdy chairs and sofas—with arms, firm backs, and seats at a height of 17 to 18 inches for ease getting up and down.

- Switch to lever-style handles instead of rotating door-knobs and faucets.

- Fix furniture such as dressers and side tables firmly in place to support body weight if someone leans on them. On furniture, switch to drawers with a single center pull, which can be opened with one hand.

- Store necessities within easy reach.

- Install oversize rocker-style light switches 32 to 36 inches high and provide remote controls for lighting.

- Adjust mattress height to 17 to 22 inches from the floor.

- Raise electrical outlets and phone jacks to 19 inches above the floor.

Beyond such steps, modern technology offers thousands of devices to help preserve human energy, strength, and capabilities while prolonging the self-sufficiency of those with limited mobility. These devices are readily available through mail-order houses and specialty shops. Many can be ordered over the telephone.

Inexpensive gadgets easily can neutralize large physical or mental handicaps. For example, does your mother find it difficult to prepare meals, reach dishes, lift pots and pans, open jars, or retrieve containers from the bottom refrigerator shelf? Levers, "reachers" with suction grippers, hand-level cabinets, large dials for stove controls, and similar clamp-on, fit-over, or screw-in replacements can solve twisting, bending, and stretching problems.

Pot stabilizers can secure saucepans to stovetops for those who can only use one hand. Sink racks can raise working levels to more comfortable heights. Loops instead of knobs can make cabinets easier to open. In the bathroom or on stairs, grab bars, chair lifts, handrails, bathtub seats, and single-stem faucets can increase convenience while reducing frustration and strain. Comb and hairbrush attachments can extend Mom's reach to compensate for limited shoulder or arm movement. Special devices can allow Dad to put on and take off his socks.

Does your wheelchair-bound father find the steps too narrow? or too steep? The doors too narrow? Are the closets and cupboards inaccessible when arthritis or a stroke inhibit a parent from lifting and reaching? A good carpenter can reduce these obstacles. When Philadelphia architect Sam O'Shiver built University Square in the late 1970s as a multipurpose complex for the elderly, low-income, and disabled, he scoured the country for the latest in barrier-free design. Since the Americans with Disabilities Act more and more housing features O'Shiver's pathbreaking ramps, walk-in showers, easy-to-reach receptacles, and accessible kitchen or closet shelves.

You can produce the same results in your parents' homes. For example, the 1994 AARP free booklet *The Do-able Re-*

newable Home: Making Your Home Fit Your Needs (AARP, 601 E St. NW, Washington, D.C. 20049) offers dozens of suggestions for stairs, bathrooms, kitchens, and entrances, and an excellent resource list.

Many states and localities make special grants to disabled residents for such home remodeling. Call the local Office on Aging to see if such funds are available. Even if they are not, remember many home modifications or devices are considered medical expenses, and are therefore tax-deductible.

There are simple things you can do to make a home safer for parents with *vision loss:*

- Mark railings, curbs, corners, and steps with bright tape.

- Reduce glare with diffuse lighting and sheer curtains (which screen bright sunlight).

- Use more warm, bright, contrasting colors; reds, oranges, and yellows are easier to see.

- Make up a personal telephone/address book with large print.

- Replace telephones with large-button versions.

For those with other disabilities, the AT&T Accessible Communication Product Center (1-800-233-1222) at 14250 Clayton Road, Ballwin, Missouri 63011, offers information and referral on inexpensive and special-needs communication devices. There are amplifiers for parents' telephone handsets and telecoils for their hearing aids to improve reception of signals from telephone receivers. Other telephone devices can help those who find it hard to move around or manipulate small objects. For example, arthritis victims find pushbutton telephones easier to operate. Cordless phones can save running to another room to pick up a phone and are especially useful for those who cannot run.

Signaling devices and alarm systems can convert sound to better perceived visual or tactile signals. For example, flashing lights and vibrating devices can amplify the ringing of a fire alarm, smoke alarm, telephone, doorbell, or alarm clock.

On the market and readily available are such other devices as writing aids for arthritics, key holders for weak fingers, and cups designed for shaky hands—as well as a door opener/closer for wheelchair patients, a non-stooping foot mop, and sewing needles with expandable eyes for easy threading. Such gadgets can be life savers or life extenders for parents. They can save you much worry and anguish, as well.

GET HELP

Suppose gadgets alone will not do, and your parents need more support to manage the hundreds of details of daily life. Who can help them when you cannot? Despite your fears, many substitutes are available; at least there are more than you think.

Do not underestimate your parents' informal network of friends, relatives, and neighbors. Encourage them to strengthen these supports with more formal community services that are also ready to help. For example, the church or alumni association or community center may have a "luncheon and activity" program of interest.

Should parents need to go out but can no longer drive, calling on a friend, an off-duty doorman, or a special senior taxi or bus or volunteer service to pick them up, can save *you* the journey. If parents are temporarily or permanently housebound, the Retired Senior Volunteer Program (RSVP) in their area may recommend projects that can be done over the telephone or at home. If parents are more frail and need daily monitoring, regular "telephone reassurance" calls by other volunteers (see p. 97) or planned arrangements with a trusted neighbor or reliable building receptionist can reduce anxiety and bring relief.

STEP 39—PREPARE A PERSONAL SUPPORT LIST WITH BACKUPS

In Part One, Step 1, you identified your parents' needs and problems. In Step 7 you developed a Personal Support List which included relatives, friends, and neighbors. In Step 21 you acquired a Directory of Community Information and Services. Now it is time to use these pieces to design a Personal Support List *including* all the backup services. Here's how:

· First, separate needs by activity. Categories might include assistance in preparing meals, dispensing medication, arranging transportation, scheduling a physical therapy program, or home repair.

· Second, using resource guides (including the research collected in your own notebook) list the names, telephone numbers, addresses, contact persons, referrals, schedules, hours of operation, and costs of services you have identified for each need—legal, medical, home health, transportation, or nutrition. This master list will include "free" help from family, neighbors, and friends; volunteer help from community programs; and paid assistance. Expand the networks by asking if those already involved can take on additional tasks or identify others who may be willing to do so. For example, if your parent is quite frail, and your family is well organized and the support network is large, you can glean some practical advice on planning a team approach to intensive caregiving from Cappy Capossela and Sheila Warnock's useful guide *Share the Care: How to Organize a Group to Care for Someone Who is Seriously Ill* (Fireside, 1995).

· Third, the AARP Booklet *Miles Away and Still Caring* recommends that you contact the key names on the support list and let them know how they can reach you, should need arise.

· Fourth, if your parents are able, perhaps they can identify resources themselves. If they cannot, and you cannot, use the "aging network" agencies to find a "case manager" or a private geriatric care manager to help draw up and coordinate this list. Again, do not rule out neighbors and friends who may want to pitch in to help out. But if your parents cannot dependably monitor their care, arrange for a backup to monitor the situation regularly.

PERSONAL SUPPORT LIST WITH BACKUP SERVICES

Activity	Resource	Contact person	Telephone number
Shopping	Local store delivery		
Meals	Meals on Wheels		
	Family		
	Restaurants		
Transport—			
Emergency			
	Ambulance		
	Taxi		
Non-emergency			
	Public transportation		
	Senior taxi (call 24 hrs in advance)		
	House bus—Schedule		
	Family/Friend/Neighbor		
	Part-time driver		
Personal care			
	Housekeeper		
	Hairdresser/Barber		
	Podiatrist/Manicurist		
	Home health agency		
	Visiting nurse		
	Neighbor/Friends/Family		

Activity	Resource	Contact person	Telephone number
Financial management			
	Bank		
	AARP volunteer		
	Accountant		
	Stock broker/Trust officer/ Pension advisor		
	Daily money manager		
Home maintenance			
	Chores/Handyman		
	Appliance service		
	Heating/Air conditioning service		
	Yardwork		
	Repair/Donations/ Consignment		
Medical			
	Doctors (by specialty)		
Medication/Prescription Buying Service			
	Local pharmacy		
	Medication monitor		
Social/Recreational			
	Library: Book/Tape/ Video rental		
	Travel: Trips/Programs		
	Clubs		
	Religious		

STEP 40—INVESTIGATE HOME HEALTHCARE

Paid "home healthcare" and its supervision is the weakest thread in the patchwork quilt of eldercare services. According to *Consumer Reports** there is little regulation of routine services, and even less quality control. What happens takes place behind closed doors, without much oversight.

The term "home healthcare" is overly broad. It covers everything from mundane chores to skilled care for acute health emergencies. It includes nursing care by registered nurses, practical nurses, or nurse's aides; physical, occupational, speech, and other therapies; nutritional guidance; hospital-type services such as chemotherapy, antibiotic therapy, breathing aides, blood testing, or heart monitoring; medically oriented social workers who help families deal with emotional, social, or economic problems; and personal care services that help with shopping, laundry, bathing, dressing, exercising, meal preparation, and housekeeping.

Medicare pays for designated health-related home care provided by a certified Home Health Care agency *after a hospitalization*. So does Medicaid. Payments are made for specific assistance by designated number of hours and number of visits.

Because of changes in the length of hospital stays, Medicare underwrites more than half of all home care provided in the nation ($15 billion in 1995). But Medicare and private health insurance rules generally favor reimbursement for institutional services. This means that it will cost your parents more to receive similar care services in the home. For example, as

*"Can Your Loved Ones Avoid a Nursing Home?" *Consumer Reports,* October 1995.

reported by the Consumer Interest Research Institute report *Home Health Care and Telecommunications,* physicians receive less Medicare reimbursement for home care than for office visits. Medications like drug-infusion therapy are reimbursed if provided in a hospital, but not if prescribed for patients in their homes. Even for custodial care—the least expensive form of home care—costs for eight-hour or twenty-four-hour shifts may equal or exceed daily rates of nursing homes.

By 1995 over 8,000 home health agencies were certified by the Health Care Financing Administration (HCFA). (If you want to check an agency's status, simply call the Medicare Hotline at 1-800-638-6833.) Home health agencies are supposed to comply with Medicare standards for staff training, competency, and similar matters. However, as *Consumer Reports* discovered,* these standards are often violated. And an equal number of home care agencies are *not certified* as Medicare providers. These agencies may operate with little oversight, except for minimal state licensing laws.

Nursing registries are another source of home care workers. They are different than certified (or noncertified) home health agencies. Registries are simply matching services that maintain rosters of available help and match them to callers' needs. Help hired through a registry usually costs less, but so is the level of supervision and quality control. Still, should your parent need help, yet not be eligible for insurance reimbursement, you may find good care through a registry. Indeed, recognizing that certified agencies generally charge up

*October 1995.

to $5 more per hour for the same aide than a registry charges, some long-term care insurance companies now reimburse policy holders needing home care for these less bureaucratic services. And in some cases, some of the same personnel are listed with both the registry and the agencies—but charge less when contacted through the registry.

Look for service that can quickly respond to your parents' shifting needs. Start with a list of the services you want the aide to perform. Be vigilant in your search for good support. Ask for word-of-mouth recommendations. The questions below were adapted from a 1986 *Washington Post* "Commentary on Homecare" column by Victor Cohn, and more recent materials downloaded from Michigan Home Health Care (see p. 132) on the World Wide Web of the internet.

1. Are you a home care agency, a registry, or an all-purpose employment agency?
2. Are you accredited, licensed or Medicare certified?
3. What qualifications, certification, experience, and training do you require of your home care workers? How do you know these requirements are met? Do you have your own training programs?
4. How long have you been in operation?
5. If my parent needs a service you do not offer, will you help me find it?
6. What are your hours? Can my parent get help every day? What about weekends, nights, or emergencies?

7. Do you perform an at-home assessment before you start? Are the family and physician consulted?

8. Do you work with the family doctor in developing a plan of care? Is a copy of the plan given to my parent and to the family? Is the plan updated as changes occur?

9. How do you monitor home care workers to make sure the plan is carried out? Are there written reports? Does a supervisor come to the home? How often?

10. Can we reach a supervisor by phone in a reasonable time when there is a complaint or question?

11. Will the same nurse (or therapist or aide) come to the home each time? Do you have a system for sending out a substitute if the worker does not show? Will you replace an aide my parent does not like?

12. How much do you charge? What will Medicare or private insurance cover? Is there a sliding scale? Do you have literature explaining your fees? What are your financial procedures?

13. Can you give three professional references (doctors, hospital personnel, or social workers)? Also the names and telephone numbers of three recent patients?

Make sure the aide is insured and the agency has workers' compensation coverage. If not, make sure your parents' homeowners' insurance is adequate to cover injuries or theft of domestic valuables. Many policies will pay only small amounts for furs, jewelry, silverware, or other items that are not specifically "scheduled."

As you have probably learned, it is often a challenge to get parents to agree to accept help at home and then to find reliable, competent, and congenial help to meet their needs. The demand for good support exceeds the supply. The advantage of using an agency is the backup support if an aide or nurse does not show up as expected. That "no show" becomes the agency's problem, not yours.

Who pays for home care? Sometimes Medicare. Sometimes Medicaid. Sometimes group health insurance. Sometimes the local Area Agency on Aging, the Veterans' Administration, or private long-term care insurance. But mostly the responsibility falls on the caretaking family. Explore your options, but be prepared to sustain much of the cost from family funds.

S E C T I O N   4

LOOKING AT HOUSING OPTIONS

The time may come when "aging in place" with available help won't work. When your parents' home is unsafe, or they are lonely, or far from their support network, or need round-the-clock support, a move may be in order—even if they can afford to hire supervised full-time staff. Keep in mind that moving can improve their quality of life and offer greater opportunities for continued independence. There are many good alternatives available besides moving in with you or into a nursing home.

STEP 41—DOWNSIZE

If their home is too large and unmanageable, your parents probably need to "downsize" to a more comfortable space. They may choose a smaller home, or an apartment, or a unit in a care living facility. Since it is not easy to shrink the contents of a life into a smaller space, be patient and show compassion. Here are some practical tips to alleviate the stress.

While discussing about the possibility of moving (a stage which may consume *years*), your parents can take preliminary steps to make an actual move far less wrenching. For some of our parents who lived during the Great Depression, or suf-

fered disruptions of World War II, the mere thought of relinquishing possessions accumulated and saved for decades
causes much anxiety. For a few, it can be overwhelming to
the point of paralysis. For others, it is just the opposite. They
relish the opportunity to make a clean sweep.

If this is an emotional minefield in your family, consider
using a third party, such as outside moving consultants or
move-in coordinators at a destination retirement community,
to help your parents' sift through personal belongings.

Depending on their style, your parents may choose to
give (or not give) treasured family heirlooms to you and
other family members during this time. This is not the moment to complicate the situation by latching onto your fa-
vorite object. Particularly one also coveted by a sibling.

If a move is planned or possible, show a lot of support.
Then go the extra mile. Have a look at all the possible and
realistic options. Work out the costs. Take time to help with
the actual move. The logistics may feel as complicated as
landing in Normandy, especially if a parent leaves one city
for another. But your help in organizing, assisting with the
sale of an existing home, disposing of unwanted household
items, arranging for post-move cleanups, and coordinating
from start to finish on moving day is absolutely necessary.
And if you can not physically be there, find someone who
can.

If your parents are less capable, you will need to make
more arrangements yourself and narrow their choices and
recommendations, but the final decision really is theirs. Only
when this approach fails—when action absolutely must be
taken, and parents cannot do it—should you decide when

and where. If other family members are involved, make sure that they agree with both the choice and the timetable. If they do not, it is very important to work out differences before the fact.

Parent Care Advisor's* suggestions for family caregivers to smooth the transition include the following.

In the months before the move:

- Consult the older person to learn what items he or she wants to take.
- Hold a family meeting. Divide moving responsibilities according to each individual's abilities, *not* their location.
- Unless competency is an issue, remember your parent has the right to choose who gets what—up to and including the home itself.
- If the home has fine art or furnishings, consider an on-site estate sale or an auction house (or storage) for special items.

In the weeks before the move:

- Measure the new location and *make sure* furniture will fit.
- List everything that will be packed and moved.

*"Planning for moving day: the practical side of downsizing," *Parent Care Advisor*, February 1995, p.8.

- Get two written bids from moving companies.

- Check with the new location about specific rules, such as availability of elevators and furniture pads during specific hours.

- Reduce clutter. Donate unwanted clothing and household items to Goodwill or the Salvation Army. Bring them in early, or arrange for them to pick up. Remember to make a list and get a receipt for tax purposes.

- Use a consignment store for better pieces of furniture, dishes, and glassware.

- Remove jewelry and small valuables separately, and store them in a safe deposit box during the move.

Finally, if there is a piano, especially a large one, hire a professional piano mover. Otherwise you may find, as we did, that hinges for the lid were tucked away in spare vacuum cleaner bags; that the piano legs were put on backwards; and that the pedals were separated in so many small pieces, it cost hours of expert labor to reassemble the parts into working order. *Nothing is saved by letting novices handle such tasks.*

FIND A BETTER PLACE

The good news is the broad range of available settings with support services for the convenience of seniors. Your first task involves gathering information on all available options. Next, you must identify the reputable operations in their community or yours. Finally you should go visit to compare services.

Unfortunately, mastering senior housing lingo is not easy. The lack of common terminology means that buzzwords and acronyms keep changing, are different in different states, and are frequently categorized under unfamiliar headings in directories. Educate yourself. Be resourceful, and keep at it! Talk to your parents, your friends, their friends and relatives. Check the Resource and Referral services mentioned in Step 21.

Look for specialized senior housing directories where your parents live. For example, the *Guide to Retirement Living* (call 1-800-394-9990 to order), lists senior housing options from aging in place, through independent living, to nursing homes for the Washington, D.C., Baltimore, and Philadelphia metropolitan areas. The *Guide* offers comparative cost and service tables for each type of senior housing available.

When exploring different options, it helps to match parents' desires for privacy with where they fit at present on an independent/assisted/dependent living spectrum, and with where they might fit six months to two years from now. When visiting potential housing, pay close attention to the presence or absence of assistive devices and improved "design for disability." This is especially relevant if the main reason for a move is to compensate for sensory, cognitive, or functional losses. If the new place is fine for today, but probably won't suit your parents in six months, keep shopping. For example, your parent now walks with a cane but with progressive osteoporosis may need a wheelchair next year (even if only for part of the day). Are there access ramps to the building and apartment doors wide enough for wheelchairs?

Ask about kitchen modifications, an emergency pull cord, accessible shelving units. Do showers have step-in entrances and seats? Who pays if these modifications are needed but not there? If these points seem obvious or minor, consider this: A 1993 study by the National Council on Disability (NCOD) reported found that "the primary reason for nursing home admissions is falls in the home or community. Equipment to prevent falls or strains such as walkers, grab-bars, reachers and appropriately located controls and switches prevented or postponed more than half of all nursing home admissions for frail elders."

The major housing options for parents in stable health include Independent Living, Assisted Living, and Continuing Care Retirement Communities, as well as nursing homes.

INDEPENDENT LIVING/SENIOR RESIDENTIAL COMMUNITIES

Available for many years, these communities integrate good security with transportation, dining services, banking, commissaries, pharmacies, and social activities. Often such senior residences are rentals or condominium townhouses or apartments. While rents can fluctuate and associated fees can go up, renting provides more flexibility than buying. They may be perfect for an independent but lonely parent. They may also suit the active parent who frequently travels and worries about security during absences. They tend to cater to a younger, healthier, and more active population of seniors.

ASSISTED LIVING

This relatively new umbrella term covers an enormous range of *nonmedical, social/residential* settings with varying levels of care, supervision, and support services. Assisted living bridges an important gap in long-term care for parents.

Assisted-living facilities are known by numerous terms with the suffix "home," or "house," or "facility," or "residence." Examples include "board and care," "homes for the aged," "domiciliary care," "half-way houses," "adult care," "foster care," "personal care," "community residence," and the old-fashioned term, "rest homes." They generally offer rental arrangements with freedom to come and go, regular house-keeping services, shared meals, and some degree of protective supervision. They may be licensed or unlicensed.

About half of the nation's estimated 70,000 assisted-living facilities are licensed under state regulations. The licensed facilities now house about 600,000 residents. But unlicensed sites serve at least an equal number of residents.

In the last ten years private developers and healthcare companies have discovered America's "aging" market. They have responded to seniors' demand for convenience and care with a new type of residence. These are apartments for the frail, but not sick, elderly. While residents live in their own apartments, rental fees include several meals a day, social activities, some transportation, some housekeeping, and minor medical care. Most of these apartment-type facilities are unlicensed because they do not fit traditional *medical* definitions of "board and care." They emphasize a more social model in which the resident and the family have much more responsibility.

An assisted-living facility may provide food and shelter for as few as two or as many as 1,400 residents. Its rates may range from $400 to $4,000 per month. It may offer a great variety of personal care, up to and including pre-arranged skilled nursing services. But hospitality and service—not healthcare—is the primary focus. This becomes crystal clear if a resident should become seriously ill or need care for more than a few weeks. In that case the resident will likely land in a hospital, with transportation politely but firmly arranged by the facility. Post-hospital care may be weak.

More than 10,000 assisted-living sites built by such companies as Sunrise, Marriott, and Hyatt are located in small towns as well as suburbs near big cities. By 1993, according to the *New York Times,* assisted living had become a $7 billion growth industry. Unlike the licensed facilities—which tend to serve a poorer population—these complexes tend to be larger, with relatively few residents who are poor or near poor.

CONSUMER BEWARE

"Good assisted living is supposed to foster independence, dignity, and privacy, a maximum level of functioning, and connections with the community," advises *Consumer Reports* (October 1995). But investigators suggest reading the fine print on costs, services, and medical options before signing any contract. They suggest asking tough questions on the availability of transportation, supplementary personal care, critical care choice, and privacy. In addition, you and your parents will want to know:

1. Can parents see their own doctors?
2. Who is in charge of medicine?
3. Suppose your parents' health fails?
4. Who decides about transfers to hospitals or other care facilities? What are your intervention points or parents' appeal rights?
5. Can parents be asked to leave? What happens if a parent's physical or mental capacity dwindles? Knowing who makes the decision, what are the factors, and whether the resident has any say is crucial.

Should your parents move to an assisted-living facility because of increasing frailty, don't expect their housing costs to be reimbursed by Medicare, private Medigap insurance, or most long-term care insurance policies, at least not yet. There may be some income support from SSI programs (see p. 168). If the trend toward community care continues, look for more support for long-term care, or tax credits for custodial caregiving. But for most "middle income" seniors— those whose annual incomes exceed roughly $25,000 per year—reimbursement benefits or tax deductions may only be available for services from a care facility *licensed* to provide medical care. An unlicensed setting may be perfect in other ways, but does not support such reimbursement.

Concerns about assisted living arise within the gray area of managing health and safety. Since our parents tend to "age in place" longer, they are moving to these sites when they are physically frailer and older. By design, assisted-living facilities offer fewer on-site supervised health services and nursing care to treat inevitable accidents and illnesses. Consequently, serious legal and moral questions for owner/operators and families center on such questions as who is at fault in case of accidental neglect, and who is responsible for the coordination and delivery of safe, secure care.

Continuous Care Retirement Communities (CCRC)

Continuous Care Communities, also known as Life Care Facilities, allow independent living in a community that supports a full range of services, from private apartments to long-term nursing care. These facilities may even include swimming pools and golf courses. A contract signed on entering describes the amount of nursing care that is covered. Upon admission, parents must be ambulatory and capable of self-care. But they are assured of housing and services for the rest of their lives, regardless of their future health or capabilities.

Continuous Care Communities are significantly more expensive than board and care homes or congregate housing. They generally require an entrance fee ranging from $50,000 to over $250,000, as well as monthly charges of $400 to $3,500. In some cases this entrance fee is refundable at death. In others it is not. Some expenses, particularly those for medical and nursing care, may be reimbursable by Medicare. Most other "custodial" costs are not.

CONSUMER BEWARE

Make sure to have a good contract lawyer or accountant check the facility's finances before signing any agreement. CCRCs are expensive, and parents may have few protections should the CCRC go out of business. The AARP's helpful pamphlet *Tomorrow's Choices* suggest asking the following questions when looking at "Life Care Facilities" as:

1. What medical costs and services does the contract cover?

2. What is the policy for transferring residents between different levels of care—and back?

3. Do fees cover all costs?

4. What is the refund policy for deposits and entrance fees? How is the refund calculated? When are your parents entitled to receive a refund? What notice must be given? When are refunds forfeited?

MOVING PARENTS INTO YOUR HOME

Contrary to what you may think, your parents may not be itching to move in with you. While several generations under one roof used to be the norm, it is a more uncommon arrangement today. An editorial in an April 1987 issue of *USA Today* noted that three or four generations under one roof has "become as rare as buggy whips and antimacassars," with only 4 percent of the over-sixty-five population living with their children. The editorial continued: "The elderly don't want to be burdens on their offspring. Their adult children say they'd rather not have Mom and Dad move in with them. Thanks to Social Security, Medicare, and medical break-throughs, the vast majority of today's senior citizens can make it on their own. And that's how they want it."

But if your parents cannot manage and good sense dictates they move in with you, you can make all the same kinds of physical changes and modifications to your home that they made (or should have made) in their own. Similarly, if parents are frailer and need more help, you can use all the services of the "aging network" to support those efforts. Even though they live with you, your parents are still eligible for such services as transportation to medical appointments, home visits by nurses and therapists, meal preparation by home health aides, and legal advice on eligibility for Medicaid. And you may be able to claim them as dependents for tax purposes.

If your parents are quite dependent, you may need to break away for a short time. Community services such as adult day care, senior centers, hospice programs, and caregiver support groups are there for people like you. These services can provide care in a therapeutic or protective environment.

For example, a local senior center or an adult day care center may be just the solution if you are working, and no one can be home with your parent. If your parent has Alzheimer's disease or is ill with cancer and you need some suggestions on how to cope while providing support, these services can be tremendously useful. If your husband wants to take a vacation, and you are afraid to leave your Mom alone, you can connect with a care facility and reserve her short-term "respite" space, or you can call a home care agency for coverage.

MOVING PARENTS TO A NURSING HOME

If your parents need full-time assistance to perform basic functions, living with you may still be possible, but too costly—in effort and stress. If this situation becomes too much to handle, the best care for your parents may be provided in a nursing home. Federal regulations, oversight, and enforcement under the 1987 Nursing Home Reform Act set standards for nursing homes receiving Medicare or Medicaid dollars. Those standards strictly limit the use of physical restraints, medications for behavior management, and involuntary transfers or discharges. They apply to those receiving chronic care as well as skilled or rehabilitative care.

Nursing homes offer twenty-four-hour access to skilled medical or intermediate care. Unlike other supportive housing, nursing homes admit residents only under a physician's order. If parents need intensive care but not hospitalization, skilled care would ordinarily be prescribed. Skilled care provides round-the-clock service by registered nurses, licensed practical nurses, and nursing assistants. It includes such services as oxygen therapy, tubes to assist breathing, and administration of intravenous fluids. Skilled care is also the only type of care generally reimbursed, under specified conditions, by Medicare.

If your parents cannot live independently, but do not need continuous intensive care, intermediate care offers such basic medical procedures as administering medicine, changing surgical dressings, giving injections, and providing range-of-motion exercises. It also offers continuous assistance with dressing, eating, and bathing. Intermediate care is for the aphasic Alzheimer's patient or bed-ridden stroke victim. Because these are not medical emergencies, Medicare rarely pays much for this type of care.

Medicaid will cover expenses after resources are exhausted. But eligibility is complicated (See Step 33). Not only must Medicaid patients qualify financially, but they must also be in a nursing home which has a "Medicaid bed" available. And many nursing homes require a waiting period as a private-pay resident before they will accept someone as a Medicaid resident.

What happens to the person who is already on Medicaid but needs to move to a nursing home or from one nursing home to another? It is not easy to find a bed. But your parents' physician or a hospital discharge planner or case manager from their Area Office on Aging can often help with placement—although the process may take time, and the destination may not be your first choice. If you are really desperate, a call to your Congressman or Congresswoman can't hurt.

There is a growing amount of literature available on choosing a good nursing home (see p. 257).

STEP 42—GET IN LINE

No matter what housing decision your parents make, as time goes by and their capabilities diminish, further changes may be necessary for which you can prepare. The reality is that almost any good place to live will have a waiting list. So visit likely spots before the last minute. If your parents are interested, take them with you. If the choice will be yours to make, place their names on these waiting lists early, to insure them a place in line. Should a vacancy in a chosen home come up before your parent is ready—you can always pass, keeping their name on the active list.

For care in nursing homes it is crucial to line up your options before the emergency. While this step may seem premature, you can save worlds of anguish and handwringing later on. Beds in good facilities are in short supply even if parents have resources to pay for them, and "Medicaid beds" will probably be restricted to current residents. If you expect your parent eventually to get on Medicaid, choose well the first time. A later switch may be quite difficult.

If the move is less drastic—for instance, from a house to an apartment in a "prime" location—the choices may also be narrow. That is true whether parents buy or rent, particularly for certain types of apartments. If your parents' goal is independent living in a retirement complex with subsidized rents, the waiting list may stretch for years. If their relocation will be from independent living to assisted living, waiting lists are also common, though the delay may be shorter.

To keep some perspective during housing discussions with your parents, emphasize to them—and keep in mind yourself—that decisions to move are usually not binding or final. Given an expected life span of fifteen to twenty years past retirement, your parents may make several moves. For example, if they are newly retired and considering giving up their co-op in Minneapolis in order to buy into a retirement community in Florida or Arizona, remind them that they do not have to make a final break at once. They may be able to rent out the Minneapolis apartment and rent their initial retirement home, joining the thousands of "snow birds" who migrate south for the winter, but return north in the summer.

It takes a while to adjust to any move, so counsel and practice patience. Just unpacking parents' boxes may take months. If it is clear the decision has turned out badly—mistakes do happen—pick up and look for a better choice. It may take some experiments to get a good fit.

PART FOUR

JUGGLING OBLIGATIONS

Juggling obligations to your job, parents, children, and friends while maintaining a cheerful temperament and putting dinner on the table is not easy, especially every day. The trick to keeping all these balls in the air is to keep your balance, concentrate, and quickly find trustworthy partners to help. Statistics indicate that with increasing life spans, juggling care for your parents with care for yourself, your children, and your job can last years. And you cannot walk away from center stage. To perform these roles successfully, you will have to focus on priorities, delegate, and—perhaps most important—keep a sense of humor.

Like it or not, unless your parents are very rich, the heaviest ball you must keep in the air is the one called "money." Money becomes a major issue if your parents need substantial attending. That is why this handbook devotes so much space to it. If you must pay for care, you will discover that caregiving is prohibitively expensive—especially if your parents need help at all times.

Even if you or family members provide most of the necessary help yourselves, you will find that effort taxing emotionally and physically as well as financially. If you live far away, you will feel the pinch with increased telephone bills, transportation costs, and work absences when a parent's decline demands monthly trips home instead of holiday visits twice a year. And emergency visits by plane or train cost significantly more than pre-planned four-day jaunts in the family car.

If the costs of caring for your parents go "off the scale" and threaten to wreck family finances, you will face even tougher decisions. You may need to choose between providing for your parents, and providing for yourself or your immediate family. The choice could be using your weekend or vacation time to provide twenty-four-hour care. But it could also mean not taking vacations, not buying a new car—or not paying your children's college tuitions. If the care period covers years, the choice may be between getting your parents financial relief through public benefit programs like Medicaid or impoverishing yourself. If you have planned for this possibility, you will know what to expect, have some sense of what you can do, and feel more in control of your life.

You will also discover that the responsibility of caring for your parents may be unevenly—perhaps unfairly—distributed. Unless you come from a family with a dozen mature married children with equally devoted spouses within three blocks from your parents—each "pitching in" by mowing the lawn, gathering groceries, cooking meals, managing the finances, submitting medical claims, visiting for tea, or taking mom or dad to the doctor—you will probably have to do a lot by yourself.

It may seem like a lot, until you share your woes with friends. There is a strong similarity among adult children describing episodes with their parents and fishermen telling tales. It seems everyone can top the previous story.

It also seems that in any family, the division of labor in caring for parents rarely is equal. Age, distance, personalities, and financial capabilities shift primary responsibilities to one adult child over another. There is often one sibling who never worries a minute and does nothing. And there always seems to be one—by choice or circumstance—who feels taken advantage of but who bears the entire burden reluctantly or gracefully. The imbalance in caregiving may be self-imposed, and the martyrdom self-fulfilling. The one who takes on the duty may shut out others perfectly willing to help, by rejecting all their offers and suggestions.

Your parents do not want to be thought of as a burden. They do not have to be, if your attitude remains positive. And the shift in responsibility does not have to be one-sided either. Sometimes kindly intervention is needed by a third party, like a doctor or a social worker, to bring about a change when families cannot or will not work together. But such changes do occur and do bring relief. If you have no siblings, spouse, or good neighbors, and your parents need a lot of help, you are allowed to grumble about having to perform a solo act. But don't think there is no one out there to listen. Professional advice and support groups are always available, and can help a lot. So can a good friend, or a sympathetic pet.

Gender is a key factor in who does what. Like it or not, in our society—and around the world—most caregiving and nurturing is still done by women. Go to any caregiving seminar in the country and look around the room. Nine of ten audience members will be women with an age range of about forty years.

You will wonder why they are there. And during the session you will find out. They are concerned about caring for their spouse, their parents, their husband's parents, their grandparents, or aging aunts, uncles, sisters, or brothers. Like you, they all have little notebooks and gather eagerly around the information table, picking up brochures that describe community services. Most have come for a specific purpose, and have lots of horror stories to tell about "the system." They attend to check out new services or learn how to work the system better. They gain strength from each other's stories. It can be an amazing experience attending these sessions, one in which common bonds are forged with strangers in minutes. You are all in the same boat.

Online support can bring help and some relief to stranded caregivers struggling with deeply emotional issues. Sometimes the anonymity helps those not comfortable sharing personal matters face-to-face.

As with all managing, your own time will be the hardest thing to juggle, especially if parent care takes a high level of effort. Some caregivers quit work completely to take on the role, while others rearrange their schedules, reduce their work hours, and take time off without pay.

If you live close by, you may find your path goes ever more frequently past your parents' house to help remove their trash, manage their bills, shovel the walk, shop for food, take them to the doctor (the bank, the supermarket), or hunt for new quarters. If you are working, you will find yourself spending job time to call agencies, doctors, and insurance providers. A study of 69 local companies conducted by the New York Business Group on Health found that work-related problems of employee-caregivers included taking time off for direct caregiving, taking time off to consult health and service agencies open only during business hours, and "excessive" telephone use, absenteeism, lateness, and unscheduled days away. "Moreover," the study concluded, "three-fifths of caregivers surveyed reported evidence of excessive stress or physical complaints, and half reported decreased productivity or quality of work performance."

Geography makes a big difference in caring for your parents. According to one recent survey, 72 percent of adult children live within minutes of their over-sixty-five parents, but 25 percent live hours away and 3 percent live days away. If your parents are like mine, and have concluded there are just two kinds of people in the world—family or everyone else—living at a distance poses problems. And as parents age—though comfortable at "home"; though surrounded by friends and memories—what they would really like is you to be near them.

For the twenty-eight percent of us whose parents do not live minutes away, caring for them—even being with them—is complicated. True, you are as near as your telephone. But reaching out to touch them electronically is not exactly the same as being there in person. Your parents may want you physically nearby, "just in case." They may want you nearby because the clock is ticking and the amount of time to spend together is running out.

What can you do when geography splits aging families? Solutions emerge slowly, sometimes painfully, based on the commitments and capabilities of everyone involved.

Some parents pull up stakes and move to be near their children, relinquishing friends and familiar surroundings. This solution will likely work best when parents' are active enough to build new relationships in their adopted homes, or realistic enough not to expect their children to fill all the hours of their day.

Others parents' prefer to stay where they are, with their adult-child moving back towards them. Still other parents will spend the year traveling the country, having long visits with each family member: wintering where it is warm, summering where it is cool. This nomad approach may work well while parents are active and mobile, but it fails when they begin to fail.

In most cases, the sibling who lives closest becomes the local firechief, putting out brushfires. More distant siblings may then assume financial or other responsibilities, provide respite, and share these tasks—however unevenly. In some families where everyone lives at a distance and the parent lives alone and is not mobile, children or close relatives take turns "riding the circuit"—arranging regular visits to "check in and check up" on parents' well-being and the quality of substitute caregivers.

Angela Heath's *Long Distance Caregiving: A Survival Guide for Far Away Caregivers* (Impact, 1993) suggests keeping a list of quick options to implement when you need to move in a hurry. For example, ask for family emergency rates, bereavement rates, and medical emergency rates from local airlines, buses, or trains. Keep their schedules in a file.

Finally, no matter how adept you may become at juggling money, siblings, and time, you will find that keeping a balanced attitude is the most difficult feat of all. You do not want—and parents do not want you—to reverse roles and become their parents. A Northern Virginia social worker, Mary Ann Carrie, has described some of the negative effects resulting from such role reversals: "The adult child feels anger that life has to end as it began . . . with dependency; anger that the parent is so self-centered; guilt over not doing more to help; guilt that you may wish them gone; grief over the loss of a strong support; and fear of abandonment. In addition there's fear that this is what the future holds for all of us. And anxiety that as the parent leaves, we are next in line. And if they're not there to help, who is?"

A parent's dependency can also arouse all the unresolved issues of past family relations. Resentments that may have simmered for years boil over when parents and adult children begin relating intensively again. Parents can manipulate childrens' feelings of guilt and sympathy. Adult children can become overbearing and domineering, taking revenge for the perceived slights they felt as children. Siblings can battle over everything from financial support to favoritism, pitching in or withdrawing support at whim. Don't think parents are not aware of these battles. They are—and it may hurt them terribly to realize they have become a cause of strife among their children. In short, caregiving itself can become a neurotic activity.

Just as you can be obsessed with caring for your children—for instance, to the point of being afraid to leave them with someone else—you can trap yourself into feeling you are the only one to care for your parents. Geriatric professionals see this often. When the job of caring for a parent becomes too great, "letting go" can be difficult. Many adult children are unable to face the fact that it is time to place a parent in a nursing home. But many more seem reluctant to use *any* public services—services their taxes and contributions support so they will be there when needed.

As you go about the business of caring for your parents, you will learn it takes time to work out these complicated relationships, and time to adjust to constantly changing situations. Certainly there are negative feelings, but there are positive ones as well. They include the feelings of moving beyond guilt and fear to acceptance and resolution; of using your energy and resilience to make life itself more meaningful.

You need to be open to suggestions, because being rigid does no good. You also need to keep looking outside for support and help—and not rejecting the help that is offered. Near or far, you don't have to do it *all*. In fact, you shouldn't even try.

This handbook is designed to help you reduce fear and stress caused by caring for your parents. It is also designed to save you time and money while doing so. By working through the tasks you have a headstart organizing your own approach to caregiving.

You have taken, or thought about taking, steps to divide tasks, reduce conflict, and promote better decisions for your family. Using the advice of others, you have adopted or considered options to protect against financial and legal catastrophe. Finally, and perhaps most importantly, you have learned that much help is available from the community outside your family.

Local, county, and volunteer programs designed to alleviate caregiver fatigue, exhaustion, and financial distress really do help. Find them. Use them. Even with these support systems, the job may not be easy. But the good news is—it's not so hard either.

A P P E N D I X   1

SELF-HELP GROUP
CLEARINGHOUSE HELPLINES

Arizona—1-800-352-3792 or 602-231-0868

Arkansas—northeast area 501-932-5555

California—San Diego 619-275-0607; San Francisco 415-921-4044;
   Sacramento 916-368-3100; Davis 916-756-8181; Modesto 209-
   558-7454

Connecticut—203-789-7645

Illinois*—708-291-0085

Indiana—northern 616-925-0594

Iowa—1-800-952-4777 or 515-576-5870

Kansas—1-800-445-0116 or 316-689-3843

Massachusetts—413-545-2313

Michigan—1-800-777-5556 or 517-484-7373

Missouri—Kansas City 816-472-HELP; St. Louis 314-773-1399

Nebraska—402-476-9668

New Hampshire—1-800-852-3388

New Jersey—1-800-FOR-MASH or 201-625-7101

New York—New York City 212-586-5770; Westchester** 914-949-
   0788 ext. 237

North Carolina—Mecklenberg area 704-331-9500

Ohio—Dayton 513-225-3004; Toledo 419-475-4449

Oregon—Portland 503-222-5555

Pennsylvania—Pittsburgh 412-261-5363; Scranton 717-961-1234

*Maintains listing of additional local clearinghouses operating within their state.
**Call Westchester only for referral to local clearinghouses in upstate New York.

South Carolina—Midlands area 803-791-9227
Tennessee—Knoxville 615-584-6736; Memphis 901-323-0633
Texas*—512-454-3706
Utah—Salt Lake City 801-978-3333
Greater Washington, D.C. 703-941-LINK

SOURCE: American Self-Help Clearinghouse, Denville, New Jersey, updated February 1996.

*Maintains listing of additional local clearinghouses operating within their state.

SENIOR HEALTH INSURANCE INFORMATION AND COUNSELING PROGRAMS

Every state, plus Puerto Rico, the Virgin Islands, and the District of Columbia has health insurance counseling programs. These programs offer consumers much useful and impartial information. Because these programs are known by different names and acronyms in various states, they may be difficult to locate. When calling the phone numbers listed below, be aware that most of the 800 numbers may work only within the state. If you have trouble finding the program in your parents state, call the ICA State Coordinator (name and telephone number listed on the right). Other sources of updated information may come from the Medicare hotline at 1-800-638-6833, or the Eldercare Locator at 1-800-677-1116. HCFA has plans to establish an Insurance Counseling Resource Center, list the various acronyms and program names, and develop a common logo for all programs.

SENIOR HEALTH INSURANCE COUNSELING PROGRAMS

STATE	PHONE	PROGRAM NAME	ACRONYM	CONTACT
Alabama	800-243-5463	Information Counseling and Assistance Program	ICA	Tenisha Jones 334-242-5743
Alaska	800-478-6065 907-562-7249	Health Insurance Counseling and Assistance Program		Deborah Taylor 907-563-5654
Arizona	800-432-4040 602-542-6595	Arizona Medigap Information and Referral Program		Joe Slattery 602-542-6446

STATE	PHONE	PROGRAM NAME	ACRONYM	CONTACT
Arkansas	800-852-5494 501-686-2940	The Seniors Insurance Network		Gloria Springer 501-686-2991
California	800-434-2222 916-323-7315	Health Insurance Counseling and Advocacy Program	HICAP	Wayne Lindley 916-323-7315
Colorado	800-544-9181 303-894-7499 x356	Senior Health Insurance Assistance Program	SHIAP	Bob Pierce 303-894-7499 x355
Connecticut	800-994-9422	Health Insurance Information Counseling and Assistance		Mimi Peck-Llewellyn 203-424-5244
Delaware	800-336-9500	Elder Information		Wendy Eaby 302-739-6266
Florida	800-963-5337 904-933-2073	Serving Health Insurance Needs of Elders	SHINE	John Venable 904-414-2060
Georgia	800-669-8387	Health Insurance Counseling Assistance and Referral for Elders	HICAP	Dawn Washington 404-657-5347
Hawaii	808-586-0100	Sage People Learning About and Under- standing the System	SAGEPLUS	Mary Dixon 808-586-0100
Idaho	800-247-4422 (SW) 800-488-5725	Senior Health Insurance Benefits Advisors	SHIBA	Kenneth Hurt 208-334-4350
Illinois	800-548-9034	Senior Health Insurance Program	SHIP	Kathy Claunch 217-782-0004
Indiana	800-452-4800	Senior Health Insurance Information Program	SHIP	Grace Chandler 317-233-5431
Iowa	800-351-4664 515-281-5705	Senior Health Insurance Program	SHIP	Kris Gross 515-242-5190
Kansas	800-432-3535	Senior Health Insurance Counseling for Kansans	SHICK	Jake Reisinger 913-296-8391
Kentucky	800-372-2973	Kentucky Benefits Counseling Program	KBCP	Valerie LaTurza 502-564-7372

STATE	PHONE	PROGRAM NAME	ACRONYM	CONTACT
Louisiana	800-259-5301 504-341-0828	Senior Health Insurance Information Program	SHIP	Rosanne Kaufman 504-342-0825
Maine	800-750-5353	Health Insurance Counseling Program in Maine		Mary Walsh 207-624-5335
Maryland	800-243-3425 410-225-1074	Senior Health Insurance and Advocacy Program	SHICAP	Michelle Holzer 410-225-1074
Massachusetts	800-882-2003 617-727-7750	Serving Health Insurance Needs of Elders	SHINE	Mary Kay Browne 617-727-7750
Michigan	800-803-7174	Medicare/Medicaid Assistance Program	MMAP	Wendi Middleton 517-373-4071
Minnesota	800-882-6262	Health Insurance Counseling Program	HICP	Angie McCollum 612-297-5459
Mississippi	800-948-3090	Mississippi Insurance Counseling and Assistance Program	MICAP	Ivory Craig 601-359-4929
Missouri	800-390-3330	Community Leaders Assisting the Insured of Missouri	CLAIM	Natalie Myers 314-893-7900 x137
Montana	800-332-2272	Montana Insurance Counseling Assistance	ICA	Gary Refslan 406-585-0773
Nebraska	402-471-2201	Nebraska Health Insurance Information Counseling and Assistance Program	NICA	Christine Curtis 402-471-4602
Nevada	800-307-4444 702-367-1218	Medicare Information, Counseling and Medicare Assistance Program	ICA	Patsy Crawford-Waite 702-367-1218
New Hampshire	800-852-3388 603-271-4642	Health Insurance Counseling Education Assistance Service	HICEAS	Tom Pryor 603-271-4701

STATE	PHONE	PROGRAM NAME	ACRONYM	CONTACT
New Jersey	800-492-8820	Counseling on Health Insurance for Medicare Enrollees	CHIME	Jack Ryan 609-292-1625
New Mexico	800-432-2080	Health Insurance Benefits Advisory Corps	HIBAC	Geralda Garcia 505-827-2080
New York (NYC)	800-333-4114 212-869-3850	Health Insurance Information, Counseling and Assistance Program	HICAP	Brendon Mooney 518-473-7259
North Carolina	800-443-9354	Seniors Health Insurance Information Program	SHIP	Carla Suitt 919-733-0111
North Dakota	800-247-0560	Senior Health Insurance Counseling Program	SHIC	Janice Cheney 701-328-2977
Ohio	800-686-1578	Ohio Senior Health Insurance Information Program	OSHIIP	Missy Brown 614-644-3575
Oklahoma	800-763-2828 405-521-6628	Senior Health Insurance Counseling Program	SHICP	Kevin Bird 405-521-6628
Oregon	800-722-4134	Senior Health Insurance Benefits Assistance	SHIBA	Joel Arlo 503-348-4018 x244
Pennsylvania	800-783-7067	"Apprise" Health Insurance Counseling and Assistance Program	APPRISE	Jack Vogelsong 717-783-8975
Puerto Rico	809-721-8590	Puerto Rico Health Insurance and Counseling Program	PRHIICP	Norma Lespier 809-721-8590
Rhode Island	800-322-2880	Senior Health Insurance Program	SHIP	Bill Doyle 401-277-2880 x220
South Carolina	800-868-9095 803-737-7500	Insurance Counseling Assistance and Referral for Elders	I-CARE	Gloria McDonald 803-737-7467
South Dakota	800-822-8804 605-773-3656	Senior Health Info and Insurance Education Program	SHINE	Mike Parker 605-773-3656

STATE	PHONE	PROGRAM NAME	ACRONYM	CONTACT
Tennessee	800-525-2816	Insurance Counseling and Assistance	ICA	Tim Watson 615-242-0438
Texas	800-252-3439	Health Information, Counseling and Advocacy Program	HICAP	Christie Fair 512-444-2727
Utah	800-439-3805 801-538-3910	Health Insurance Information Program	HIIP	Sally Brown 801-538-3910
Vermont	802-828-3302	Health Insurance Counseling and Assistance Program	HICA	Camille George 802-241-2400
Virginia	800-552-3402	Virginia Insurance Counseling and Advocacy Project	VICAP	M. T. Grund 804-225-2801
Virgin Islands	809-774-2991	—		Iris Bermudez 809-773-6449
Washington	800-397-4422	Seniors Health Insurance Benefits Advisors	SHIBA	Joan Lewis 206-654-1833
Washington, D.C.	202-676-3900	Health Insurance Counseling Project	HICP	Sue Anderson 202-676-3900
West Virginia	800-642-9004 304-558-3317	Senior Health Insurance Network	SHINE	Barbara Reynolds 304-558-3317
Wisconsin	800-242-1060	Medigap Helpline and Employer Benefit Specialists		Glen Silverberg 608-267-3201
Wyoming	800-856-4398	Wyoming Senior Health Insurance Information Program	WSHIIP	Jade Kauffman 307-856-6880

SOURCE: Telephone numbers from final proof of *1996 Medicare Handbook*, ICA State Coordinator Listing, from ICA Grants Program, Health Care Financing Administration, Baltimore, Maryland (May 1996). Program Names and Acronyms, survey of Health Insurance Counseling Programs, United Seniors Health Cooperative, Washington, D.C. (November 1995).

ELDERCARE INTERNET ADDRESSES

RESOURCES

INTERNET AND E-MAIL RESOURCES ON AGING
   http://www.aoa.dhhs.gov/aoa/pages/jpostlst.html
ADMINISTRATION ON AGING HOME PAGE
   http://www.aoa.dhhs.gov
DIRECTORY OF WEB AND GOPHER AGING SITES
   http://www.aoa.dhhs.gov/aoa/webres/craig.htm or
   http://www.aoa.dhhs.gov/aoa/pages/loctrnew.html

GENERAL SITES FOR CAREGIVERS AND SENIORS (ALPHABETICAL)

BLACKSBURG ELECTRONIC VILLAGE SENIOR INFORMATION (BEV)
   http://www.bev.net/community/seniors
CAREGIVERS
   http://www.sfgate.com/examiner/caregivers series
ELDERCARE WEB.
   http://www.ice.net/~kstevens/ELDERWEB.HTM
INSTITUTE OF GERONTOLOGY
   http://www.iog.wayne.edu
SENIOR.COM
   http://www.senior.com

SELECTED STATE AND COMMUNITY RESOURCES ON THE INTERNET

CAREGIVERS RESOURCE GUIDE

http://www.sfgate.com/examiner/caregivers/resources/national.html

CHICAGO DEPARTMENT ON AGING

http://www.ci.chi.il.us/WorksMart/Aging

CLEVELAND FREENET

Alzheimer's Disease Support Center (ADSC)

Modem Connection: Telnet to: freenet-in-b.cwru.edu

DIRECTORY OF ST. LOUIS RESOURCES FOR SENIORS

http://www.riversidepavillion.com/dirorg.html

PRINCETON UNIVERSITY ELDERCARE CONTACT RESOURCE GUIDE

http://www.princeton.edu/Main/elder.html

SPECIFIC TOPICS (ALPHABETICAL)

Coping skills

EMOTIONAL SUPPORT GUIDE

http://asa.ugl.lib.umich.edu/chdocs/support/emotion.html

Disability

1. NETWATCH TOP TEN—NET ACCESS FOR DISABLED

http://.pulver.com/netwatch/topten

2. DISABILITY RESOURCES ON THE INTERNET

http://disability.com

Elder law

KANSAS ELDER LAW NETWORK (KELN)

http://ukanaix.cc.ukans.edu/~webmom/keln_main.html

Government information

1. FEDWORLD INFORMATION NETWORK

http://www.fedworld.gov

2. LIBRARY OF CONGRESS

http://www.loc.gov

Health care

1. HYPERDOCMED

    http://ncbi.nlm.nih.gov/cgi-bin/medline?aging+%26+theory

    http://www.nlm.nih.gov/

2. SEARCH ENGINE: YAHOO—HEALTH

    http://www.yahoo.com/Health

Alzheimer's disease and dementia

1. ALZHEIMER'S DISEASE AND DEMENTIA

    http://www.biostat.wustl.edu/alzheimer/

    gopher://gopher.ardc.wustl.edu/

2. ALZHEIMER PAGE—WWW LINKS ON AGING AND DEMENTIA

    http://www.biostat.wush.edu/ALZHEIMER/submit.html

3. ALZHEIMER'S ASSOCIATION (U.S.)

    http://www.alz.org

Home care

1. IN HOME HELP—MICHIGAN HOME HEALTH CARE

    http://www.traverse.com/health/mhhc/home.html

2. NATIONAL ASSOCIATION FOR HOME CARE (NAHC)

    http://www.nahc.org/

Housing

1. SENIOR SITES

    http:www.seniorsites.com

2. "GUIDE TO CHOOSING A NURSING HOME"

    gopher://gopher.gsa.gov:70/00/staff/pa/cic/health/nursehme.txt

Insurance

NATIONAL COMMITTEE FOR QUALITY ASSURANCE (MANAGED CARE)

    http://www.ncqa.org

Long-term care

AMERICA'S HOUSE CALL NETWORK

    http.www.housecall.com

Medicare

HEALTH CARE FINANCING ADMINISTRATION

    http://hcfa.gov/medicare/medicare.html

Medication
PharmInfo Net
   http://pharminfo.com/pin__hp.html
Social Security
Social Security Online
   http://www.ssa.gov/programs/programs__intro.html

SAMPLE AGING RELATED DISCUSSION GROUPS/LISTSERVS

Gerinet

To send a message or reply to the list after you are a sub-scriber use: GERINET@UBVM.CC.BUFFALO.EDU
   http://tile.net/tile/cgi-bin/gerinet.html

BULLETIN BOARD SYSTEMS

Agenet

Call the BBS at 1-800-989-2243 (8 bits and 1 stop bit).

Give name and select a password. Menus will guide you through online session.

COMMERCIAL ONLINE SERVICES

1. America Online (1-800-827-9948)
2. CompuServe (1-800-848-8199)

SUGGESTED RESOURCES AND SOURCE MATERIALS

How to Care for Your Parents mentions some of the better known national organizations and agencies dealing with the many issues related to caregiving. To locate the name and telephone number of an organization by topic, please refer to the listing of Community Resources on p. 77. For example, "Caregiver Support" gives information about self-help organizations like Children of Aging Parents and the Well Spouse Foundation. "Home Improvement Services" gives the toll-free number of ABLE-DATA, the National Rehabilitation Information Center on assistive equipment, devices, and furniture to help the disabled.

The Eldercare Locator is the best place to start gathering information on local Area Agencies on Aging services. Call 1-800-677-1116 for information.

In addition, there are a growing number of organizations that offer services to help caregivers. Here are just a few:

Children of Aging Parents (CAPS) Levittown, Pennsylvania (phone: 1-800-227-7294). offers telephone counseling, a bimonthly newsletter and publications on a variety of caregiver issues such as "How to Find Resources in Your Area."

Family Caregiver Alliance, San Francisco, California (phone 1-415-434-3388). http:www.caregiver.org. An information, education, and service agency for families and professionals caring for adults with cognitive disorders such as Alzheimer's disease, stroke, head injury, and Parkinson's disease. Free fact sheets on community based serves, statistics, local services, and other publications.

The Rosalynn Carter Institute for Human Development, Americus, Georgia (phone: 1-912-928-1234).

Information on self help organizations can be found in *The Self-Help Sourcebook: Finding & Forming Mutual Aid Help- Groups,* Fifth Edition, eds. Barbara J. White and Edward H. Madara, New Jersey, 1995. $9.00 (available from American Self-Help Clearinghouse at phone: 1-201-625-7101).

FOR GENERAL INFORMATION

Answers: For Adult Children Of Aging Parents is a bimonthly magazine. based in Richmond, California. Yearly subscription rate $21.95. Call 1-800-750-2199 or visit the Website at http:www.service.com/answers/cover.html.

Parent Care Advisor's monthly newsletter offers timely tips and resources for caregivers. The subscription rate is $95 for 12 issues. (For a free copy call 1-800-341-7874 ext. 347.)

Caregiver's Guide: Helping Older Friends and Relatives with Health and Safety Concerns. Carolyn Robb and Janet Reynolds. Boston: Houghton Mifflin, 1992. $13.95.

Helping Yourself Help Others: A Book for Caregivers. Rosalynn Carter with Susan K. Golant. New York: Random House, 1996. $14.00.

Long Distance Caregiving: A Survival Guide for Far Away Caregiving. Angela Health. San Luis Obispo, CA: Impact Publishers, 1993. $9.95.

Taking Care of Aging Family Members: A Practical Guide. Wendy Lustbader and Nancy R. Hooyman. New York: The Free Press, 1994. $14.95.

FINANCIAL INFORMATION

Long Term Care: A Dollars and Sense Guide. Washington, D.C.: United Seniors Health Cooperative, 1993. $8.50 plus S&H. (Available from United Seniors. Call 1-202-393-6222.)

HEALTH

Complete Guide to Aging and Health, Mark E. Williams, M.D. American Geriatric Society. New York: Harmony Books, 1995. $26.00 plus $5.70 S&H). (Available from AGS. Call 1-800-677-9944.)

How We Die: Reflections on Life's Final Chapter. Sherwin B. Nuland. New York: Vintage Books, 1995. $13.00.

36 Hour Day: A Family Guide to Caring for Persons with Alzheimer's Disease, Related Dementing Illness, and Memory Loss in Later Life. Second Revised Edition. Nancy L. Mace and Peter V. Rabins. Baltimore, MD: Johns Hopkins Press, 1991. $11.95.

HOME IMPROVEMENT–ASSISTIVE DEVICES

Enrichments Product Catalog "Products to Enhance Your Life." Everything from non-tie shoelaces to pedal exercisers that go in front of a chair. Bolingbrook, Illinois. (Call 1-800-323-5547 for a free catalog.)

"Gadgets, Gizmos, and Thingamabobs: The Wonderful World of Self-Help" Video and Resource Directory. Center for the Study of Aging. Washington, D.C.: Serif Press. Call 202-737-4650.

"The Do-Able Renewable Home: Making your Home Fit Your Needs. 1994. (D12470). AARP Fulfillment (EE09040), 601 E. St. NW, Washington, D.C. 20049. Free.

HOUSING

The American Association of Homes and Services for the Aging (AASA) offers several free pamphlets. Phone: 1-202-783-2242 to request: "Assisted Living"; "Choosing a Nursing Home"; "Continuing Care Retirement Communities"; or "Housing Care Options."

The Guide to Retirement Living. Annual Guides detailing specifics on numerous senior housing options available in Washington, D.C., Baltimore, Maryland and Philadelphia, Pennsylvania. McLean VA: Douglas Publishing. For a FREE copy, call 1-800-394-9990.

INSURANCE

The Health Insurance Association of America (HIAA) offers various consumer publications on long-term care insurance. Write HIAA at P.O. Box 41455, Washington, D.C. 20018.

MEDICARE

The Health Care Financing Administration offers valuable publications and audiotapes on Health Insurance and Medicare. Call the Social Security Administration: 1-800-772-1213, or the Medicare Hotline between 8 A.M. and 8 P.M. eastern time, M–F at 1-800-638-6833. Request free copies of the following publications: *Your Medicare 1995 Handbook; 1995 Guide to Health Insurance for People with Medicare;* and *Medicare and Managed Care Plans.*

LEGAL

"Shape Your Health Care Future with Health Care Advance Directives." To get a copy, write AARP–AD, P.O. box 51040, Washington, D.C. 20091. $2.00.

VIDEO

Aging Parents: The Family Survival Guide. 2 videos plus guide. San Francisco, CA: SyberVision, 1996. (To order, call 1-800-456-0678.)

Visit your local libraries and large bookstores. Look in the Family, Financial, and Self-Help sections. Write the Center for Books on Aging, a division of Serif Press Inc. at 1331 H St. NW, Washington, D.C. 20005 or call them at 1-202-737-4650 or 1-800-221-4272. The Center's free catalog of more than 2,000 titles, videos, and audio tapes from more than 300 publishers features a buying services for professionals, libraries, aging agencies, and individuals.

LIVING WILL AND HEALTH CARE PROXY SAMPLES

LIVING WILL

To: My Family, my Physicians, my Lawyer, any Medical Facility in whose care I happen to be, any Individual who may become responsible for my Health Affairs, and All Others Whom It May Concern:

I, being of sound mind and over 18 years of age, hereby issue a directive, which I intend to be legally binding, **which shall become effective at some future time, only under the following circumstances:**

1. When I become unable to make my own decisions or express my wishes; *AND*

2. CHOOSE ALL THAT YOU WANT TO APPLY

❑ If I have a terminal illness; and/or

❑ I am permanently unconscious; and/or

❑ If extraordinary life support procedures or "heroic measures" would be medically futile; and/or

❑ Under the following circumstances (Please specify, for example, dementia, severe neurological illness or other permanent disabling condition to which you want this Directive to apply):

_____

_____

_____

_____

Then I direct that my dying not be unreasonably prolonged; *AND*

CHOOSE *ONE*

❏ I wish to have COMFORT CARE ONLY, which is directed only toward relieving pain and suffering, regardless of the progress of my disease.

❏ I want CONSERVATIVE CARE, which is usual treatment (such as antibiotics) *but not* extraordinary treatment (such as cardiopulmonary resuscitation, mechanical ventilation, kidney dialysis, etc.).

OPTIONAL: I wish to make additional directives (about life support equipment or other matters):

_____

_____

_____

_____

PLEASE NOTE: If, at some future time, you cannot make decisions for yourself, New York State law prohibits withholding artificial nutrition and hydration from you, unless you have already made your wishes known.

If I cannot eat or drink enough because of my irreversible medical conditions: (❏ I DO / ❏ I DO NOT) want artificial nutrition (intravenous or tube feeding) and hydration (intravenous fluids).

In the absence of my ability to give directions regarding the aforementioned life sustaining procedures, it is my intention that this directive shall be honored as the final expression of my legal right to refuse medical treatment and to accept the consequences of such refusal.

I understand the full importance of this directive and I have signed it after thorough consideration of the nature and consequences of my refusal of such extraordinary life support procedures, including their benefits and disadvantages. This directive is in accordance with my strong convictions and beliefs and is made freely without any inducement or coercion from any person or institution.

_____   _____
SIGNATURE   DATE

I hereby certify that I am over 18 years of age and that I have witnessed the above declarant's signature.

_____   _____
WITNESS   WITNESS

_____   _____
PRINTED WITNESS NAME   PRINTED WITNESS NAME

_____   _____
DATE   DATE

HEALTH CARE PROXY

I, _____ hereby appoint the following person as my HEALTH CARE AGENT, to make any and all health care decisions for me except for any restrictions I have noted below. This Proxy shall take effect when and if I become unable to make my own health care decisions.

_____
HEALTH CARE AGENT NAME   PHONE

_____
ADDRESS

_____
ALTERNATE HEALTH CARE AGENT NAME   PHONE

_____
ADDRESS

Optional instructions or limitations on the Health Care Agent's authority, if any:

_____

_____

_____

_____

Unless I revoke it, this Proxy shall remain in effect indefinitely. (Or until the date or condition stated below, if any.)

_____

_____

PLEASE NOTE: If, at some future time, you cannot make decisions for yourself, New York State law prohibits your Health Care Agent from making decisions about withholding artificial nutrition and hydration from you, unless you have already made your wishes known.

If I cannot eat or drink enough because of my irreversible medical conditions: (❑ I DO / ❑ I DO NOT) want artificial nutrition (intravenous or tube feeding) and hydration (intravenous fluids).

_____   _____
SIGNATURE   DATE

_____
ADDRESS

I hereby certify that I am over 18 years of age, and that the person who signed this Proxy appeared to do so willingly and free from duress and that he or she signed (or asked another to sign for him or her) this Proxy in my presence.

_____   _____
WITNESS   WITNESS

_____   _____
PRINTED WITNESS NAME   PRINTED WITNESS NAME

_____   _____
DATE   DATE

KEYWORD INDEX (ACRONYMS)

NOTES